HEALTH AND LIFESTYLE SURVEY

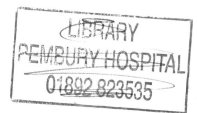

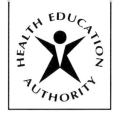

THE HEA HEALTH AND LIFESTYLE SURVEY

A report on the secondary analysis of a national dataset of health-related knowledge, attitudes and behaviour

Contributors

Barrie Margetts   Senior Lecturer
Viv Speller   Senior Lecturer
Rachel Thompson   Senior Research Fellow
The Wessex Institute for Health Research and Development,
University of Southampton

Dominic McVey   Head of Research
Health Education Authority

Katherine Oldfield, Liz Rogers, Jane Royle and Nicola Woodward
(The Wessex Institute for Health Research and Development) contributed to
the organisation of workshops and drafts of earlier versions of this report.

Rhiannon Barker (Health Education Authority) and Rosemary Pope
(formerly HEA) deserve a special thank you for their contribution to the
design and management of the survey.

The HEA would like to thank all the respondents who consented to take
part in this survey and gave so generously of their time.

WA 900

HEALTH
LIFESTYLE
ATTITUDE TO lth
SURVEY

ISBN 0 7521 0989 8

First published 1998

Health Education Authority
Trevelyan House
30 Great Peter Street
London SW1P 2HW

Typeset by Wayzgoose
Printed and bound by Antony Rowe Ltd.

Contents

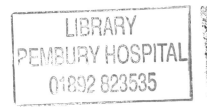

•

Tables

4. Nutrition

5. Sexual health

6. Association between nutrition, smoking and sexual health

Figures

3. Smoking

4. Nutrition

5. Sexual health

6. Association between nutrition, smoking and sexual health

Foreword

The HEA has funded several Health and Lifestyles surveys during the 1990s – the 1992 Health and Lifestyle survey, the 1995 Health Education Monitoring Survey and the 1993 Black and Minority Ethnic Group survey. All have been widely distributed and well received by researchers and programme makers as valuable sources of data on health-related knowledge, attitudes, beliefs and behaviour. A follow-up survey to the Health and Lifestyles survey of 1992 was conducted during 1993 and 1994 and rather than produce a standard descriptive report, the results were reported through a range of different media to inform the development and evaluation of health education programmes.

For a variety of reasons, mainly related to the availability of time and money, much of the data generated from national surveys, emanating from many government departments, is not subjected to the in-depth multivariate analysis which can often reveal useful and sometimes surprising insights into human motivations and behaviour. With this in mind the HEA revisited the data generated by the 1993 Health and Lifestyle survey and commissioned Wessex Institute of Public Health to work with the HEA to go beyond the familiar descriptive analysis expected from large national surveys of this nature. In parallel with this exercise, three regional workshops (Southampton, London and Birmingham) were convened with researchers and purchasers from the NHS to collect their views on the type of analyses that would be valuable and how these could most usefully be presented in a final report. In this report basic descriptive statistics are revisited to set the context for the multivariate analysis on smoking, diet and sexual health which divides the population into key demographic clusters. Finally, using this cluster analysis the associations between poor diet, smoking and risky sexual behaviour are examined.

This report describes one way of looking at this data and there are many more varied analyses, which can be performed. The HEA Research Directorate is committed to exploring existing data sets to ensure that full value is gained from these large studies, and to help achieve this we are currently conducting a number of secondary analysis projects. To help researchers gain a fuller picture of the data available in Britain, the HEA have also produced a CD ROM comprising information on national surveys of health and lifestyles, funded by the HEA and others. Researchers are welcome to perform their own analysis on any of the HEA national datasets to help us all develop a greater understanding of our rich and varied attitudes and behaviours.

Dominic McVey
Head of Research, Health Education Authority

1. Summaries of key points

Smoking

This survey demonstrates the continuing decline in smoking rates; 29% of men and 27% of women were smokers in 1993. Smoking rates are highest for young women aged 20–24 years and men aged 25–34 years; for women who are separated or divorced, and for men and women who live together. Smoking prevalence is also high for both men and women who have no formal qualifications and are in manual jobs.

Half of all current smokers live in rented accommodation, half of current smokers are on income support or are unemployed, and half live in households with at least one other smoker. Over half of single mothers smoke, and over half of people living in younger, low-income families are smokers. Heavy smokers are more likely to be men, manual workers, living in the North of England or in younger, low-income families.

Women are increasingly starting to smoke at younger ages. Manual workers, and respondents in younger, low-income families are more likely to start smoking before the age of 16 years. The older men and women were when they started to smoke, the more likely they are to be able to stop. Lighter smokers are also more likely to give up. Most ex-smokers gave up between 25 and 34 years of age. Women in manual occupations, those living with a smoker, and smokers in younger, low-income families are less likely to try to stop, and to succeed.

Smokers and non-smokers are generally permissive in their attitudes towards allowing visitors to smoke in their homes. Most current smokers feel they should not smoke in restaurants, but fewer younger smokers agree. Smokers in younger, low-income families and older, less-educated smokers are more likely than others to ignore smoking bans in public. There seems to be wide acceptance of not smoking near babies, children and pregnant women; but there is less acceptance by older people and those in manual occupations of the need for women to stop smoking in pregnancy.

Older smokers, and those who smoke less than twenty a day are more likely to think that smoking is not having an effect on their health. Short-term health effects such as breathlessness and cough were acknowledged more frequently than the risk of cancer or heart disease. People who have never smoked, and younger people, are more aware of the effect of passive smoking on other people's health. About half of parents with children under 16 thought that parental smoking made children more likely to smoke. Smoking parents appear not to recognise the impact of their smoking on the likelihood of their children smoking. One-third of fathers who smoke, and one-fifth of mothers, thought their children would be more likely to smoke; while one in six fathers who smoked, and one in four mothers, thought that their children would be *less* likely to smoke.

Nutrition

Most people thought that they knew something about how to reduce their risk of heart disease, but fewer knew about how people could reduce their risk of diabetes and stroke; very few knew what people could do to prevent osteoporosis. The benefits of exercise in reducing the risk of osteoporosis were known by only a few. In general women were more likely than men to believe that people could reduce their risk of disease, and those who were middle-aged and educated were more likely to believe that risk could be reduced than those in younger, low-income families.

Although respondents felt reasonably confident explaining about fats in general, most were not confident that they could explain about types of fat, or E numbers. Those who were middle-aged and educated were more likely to correctly identify foods high in fat than those who were older and less educated. There were some inconsistencies in people's knowledge about the fat content of margarine compared with butter, many incorrectly thought margarine was low in fat and even those who felt confident in their knowledge of fats were confused about margarine.

Nearly half of the respondents felt well informed about cholesterol and most had correct knowledge about a series of statements about cholesterol. There were considerable demographic group differences in knowledge about cholesterol and the saturated fat content of foods; those who felt well informed about saturated fats were more likely to be correct, and non-manual subjects were generally better informed than those in manual occupations.

Many people from all socio-demographic clusters are eating 'less healthy' diets, but this was highest for those in younger, low-income families where two-thirds were eating less healthy diets.

Cost is a major factor in influencing where people shop and what they buy. The socio-demographic differences indicated the need for a more targeted approach to improving dietary practices which takes account of people's income and access to shops.

The men who are most likely to benefit from dietary change are manual workers who are least likely to eat lunch in a workplace canteen, one-half eating a packed lunch from home. The reverse is true for women, with more in non-manual occupations eating a packed lunch.

Based on self-reported data, one-third of women aged 16–19 years are underweight, and 14% of men and women aged 45–54 years are obese. In general more manual workers are obese than non-manual workers.

It appears that about one-third of men and women are confused about healthy eating. Those that ate a more healthy diet were more likely to think that fresh fruit and vegetables were part of a healthy diet, and that eating more fruit and vegetables could reduce the risk of heart disease. Many people have changed their diet over the last three years, although younger people in manual occupations have made the least change.

The demographic profiles were a strong determinant of eating patterns, perceptions about a healthy diet, and barriers to change to a healthy diet. The younger, low-income families, and older less educated groups are less likely to eat a healthy diet or to have changed their diet in the last three years. They are more likely to believe that healthy diets are a fashion and expensive, and to have cost as a limiting factor in where to shop and what to buy.

Sexual health

The age at which young men and women first have intercourse is decreasing, and those in manual occupations are more likely to have their first sexual intercourse under 16 years of age. Those in the socially disadvantaged cluster (in rented accommodation, on benefits, single parents and manual workers), are more likely to have had two or more partners in the last year. Men and women who describe themselves as being in 'steady' relationships (but not married) are also more likely to have had two or more partners in the last year.

Two-thirds of men and women think sex education should be provided mainly by parents, and that parents should be included by schools in sex education, although women were more likely to think this than men. Most people think that factual topics about sex and contraception should be included in sex education, but women would like to see more about feelings, emotions and personal choice in school sex education. One-quarter of men and women thought that it was very important to include education about homosexuality and lesbianism in school sex education lessons.

Most men and women do not think that showing of television adverts for AIDS and condoms should be restricted to after 9 pm.

Most men and women do not think that they have adequate knowledge of emergency contraception, recognising the symptoms of sexually transmitted diseases, or having an HIV test.

Less than a fifth of women, and slightly fewer men, report not using any contraceptives the last time they had sex. Overall one-fifth of men and women did not use any contraceptives the first time that they had sex, but for those whose first intercourse was more recent (between 1991 and 1993) this had reduced to 5–6%, demonstrating the success of safer sex campaigns. Barrier methods of contraception are most popular at first intercourse and the

3

use of condoms is increasing with about three-quarters of men and women using condoms the first time between 1991 and 1993. However, people in the 'worse-off' demographic cluster are less likely to use contraception at first intercourse than those who are 'better off'.

Women, whether or not they are in steady relationships, tend to change over time to using the pill as a method of contraception; but men who are not in steady relationships continue to use condoms. When asked what would stop them using condoms, most men and women said they would forget to carry them, or would get 'carried away in the heat of the moment'; in particular people not in a steady relationship also said that they would be likely to forget to carry condoms.

An HIV risk score was computed from the number of sexual partners in the last year, and use of condoms. This indicated that 5% of men and 3% of women are at high risk of contracting HIV; younger and manual workers, and those in the 'worse-off' cluster were at higher risk. Of those who had two or more partners in the last year, women and older respondents were also at higher risk. There is also a potentially neglected higher-risk group of older men, who are either coming out of steady relationships or having affairs, who are not using condoms.

Men and women at higher risk of HIV were more likely to forget to carry condoms, and to get 'carried away'. All factors that are likely to stop condom use, including cost, were higher for the 'worse-off' group.

About three-quarters of men and women felt that they were not at all at risk of HIV or STDs, and those at higher and moderate risk of HIV do underestimate their personal risk. Less than half of those at higher risk think that their sex life is not at all risky. About a quarter of men and a fifth of women overall are worried about getting HIV, but more people in the 'worse-off' group are worried and are in fact at higher risk of HIV. Very few people have sought voluntary testing for HIV and this does not differ by risk group.

Associations between nutrition, smoking and sexual health

Smokers eat less healthily than never or ex-smokers, smokers in the North and Midlands eat less healthily than smokers in the South; and smokers in younger low-income families and the older less-educated group eat less healthily. There appears to be a relationship between smoking cessation and changing to a healthier diet.

There is some indication that persons with a higher sexual health risk as determined by HIV risk score are more likely to be smokers, to eat a less healthy diet and are less likely to change to a healthier diet.

Those who have never smoked or have given up and who have a low HIV risk score are more likely to eat a healthy diet than smokers at higher HIV risk.

2. Methods, and characteristics of the population

This chapter describes the methods used to collect data in the present study, the approach used in analysing the data, and a demographic profile of respondents.

Methodology

The sampling procedure and fieldwork were carried out by MORI between May and September 1993 in England only.

Sampling procedure

MORI conducted a random probability survey, using a nationally representative sample of 386 census enumeration districts which were selected at random within England, for persons aged between 16 and 74 years of age. The probability of selection within each enumeration district was proportional to the population within each enumeration district aged between 16 and 74 years of age. Within each enumeration district 65 addresses were drawn at random from the Small Users' Postcode Address file. Twenty-five of these addresses were drawn to form a booster sample of 16- to 24-year-old respondents. The sample was stratified by the eight NHS regions.

A letter was sent to each address included in the survey to explain the purpose of the survey and to inform people that a MORI interviewer would be calling at their address. The sample addresses were screened by interviewers and those which were identifiable as invalid (non-residential, vacant, demolished, etc.) were eliminated from the sample. Addresses were screened for multiple households and if necessary a Kish grid (Kish, 1965) was used to select one of the households resident at the address. The principles of a Kish grid are described in further detail in the appendix to this chapter.

Selected households were then screened by interviewers to obtain a listing of all adults eligible to take part in the survey; that is those aged between 16 and 74 years of age in the main sample or between 16 to 24 years at the booster address normally resident at the address. Households containing only people over 75 years of age, and in the booster households those not aged between 16 and 24 years of age, were eliminated from the study.

The required sample for this study was 5550 subjects; 4550 people aged between 16 and 54 years of age (including 550 from the boosted sample for

16- to 24-year-olds), and 1000 aged between 55 and 74 years of age. The proportion of subjects over 55 years of age was higher than that found in the population at large and it was therefore necessary to screen out some of the older people identified. One in two households containing only 55- to 74-year-old persons were eliminated from the sample. In households containing both 16- to 54-year-old persons and 55- to 74-year-old persons, each younger person was given twice as great a chance of being selected as an older person. In households where there was more than one potential respondent, the intended respondent was selected using a Kish grid.

Response rate

The initial sampling strategy identified 21 755 addresses, which after checking for invalid addresses (vacant , demolished etc.) was reduced to 19 617 which were contacted by letter. Of these addresses interviewers were able to screen households at 14 822 addresses (76% of the 19 617 contacted); 2416 households refused, and 2379 households could not be contacted even after four attempts. Of the 14 822 households screened by the interviewer: 5064 households were excluded because they contained no household member aged between 16 and 24 years of age; 1080 were excluded because all the residents were over 75 years of age, and 791 households were excluded as part of selecting only one in two households where subjects only aged between 55 and 74 years of age were resident; leaving 7887 addresses identified with a person who was eligible to be interviewed. Of the 7887 eligible subjects: 1419 refused to be interviewed (18%); 601 (8%) non-contacts even after repeated calls (minimum of four) at the house; 314 (4%) were not interviewed because they were too ill or had moved away since the original screening. Interviews were conducted with 5553 respondents, 70% of the 7887 eligible subjects. Response rate for the self-completed questionnaire was 84%.

Data collection

Data were collected from the respondent, about the respondent, not the head of the household. All respondents completed a face-to-face interview covering their (and their households) demographic characteristics, smoking and nutrition. Respondents aged between 16 and 54 years of age were handed a self-completion questionnaire covering questions about sexual health; respondents were asked to complete the questionnaire and place it in an envelope and return it to the interviewer who was present while the questionnaire was completed; the interviewer did not check the completeness of the questionnaire with the respondent.

All interviewers were trained prior to undertaking the interviews and were given a detailed manual for guidance.

Data on food consumption was obtained using the DINE questionnaire, which had been calibrated previously (Roe et al., 1994). MORI interviewers were instructed to follow the format exactly as specified; for example they were asked to find out about the one type of bread respondents ate most often. They were not allowed to state two types of bread eaten equally often.

Data coding and error checking procedures used

A full manual edit was carried out on every interviewer's first day of work on the survey. Throughout the survey, additional visual edit checks were carried out on key questions for all returned questionnaires. During data entry, checks were made for accuracy and completeness of coding. For open-ended questions coding frames were developed in consultation with the HEA.

Design of questionnaire

The interview took about an hour to complete. Where respondents were not the head of the household, and where they also had a partner, they were asked to provide demographic details about these people. In the present report we have only presented data on the respondent, as the data on the head of the household was incomplete.

Questions on health status and smoking were the same as those used in the 1992 survey. Other questions were developed by the HEA after consultation with relevant experts. Questionnaires were piloted in 10 sampling points, with 50 interviews.

Weighting

The survey data were weighted in two ways: by household size – each respondent received a weight proportional to the number of adults in the household, to correct for the fact that MORI only interviewed one adult per household, thereby lessening the chances of selection for adults in larger households. Data were also weighted by age within gender within NHS regions, using census estimates (see Appendix B).

Analysis

Introduction

Before the data were analysed subjects' responses to groups of questions were checked for internal consistencies and any obvious coding errors such as, for example, 'never smokers' having 'numbers of cigarettes smoked'. The analysis proceeded in a stepped progression: initial simple exploratory analyses by gender were followed by more in-depth analyses of responses by age, occupation, marital status, and region of residence. For some analyses where the numbers of subjects in each stratum were small, age, occupation and regions were grouped: for age into three groups (16–24, 25–44 and 45–74 years); regions into two groups (north – Northern & Yorkshire, Trent, West Midlands and North West; South – Anglia and Oxford, North Thames, South Thames; and South and West); and for occupation into two groups (manual and non-manual).

All tables present weighted data. Data were weighted by a factor which took into account age, gender, region and household type to ensure that any pooled estimate reflected the general population estimate. Unweighted figures, without correcting for age, gender, region and household type, would not reflect national data as younger males and females would be overrepresented.

Statistical summaries and analyses have been kept relatively simple, the aim of the analysis was to explore those factors which influenced people's smoking, nutrition and sexual health knowledge, attitudes and behaviour, together with an analysis of the interaction between these factors. Where percentages do not add up to 100 this was due to rounding of responses. Because the sample size for this study was large, most basic comparisons of the whole population when broken down by gender were statistically significantly different.

Given the large number of comparisons presented in this report it is likely that a number of statistically significant associations will have occurred by chance alone. The analyses undertaken assumed a simple random sample, which was not the case in the present study, so that the significance tests based on the present data are approximate.

Statistical significance does not automatically equate to biological significance and caution should be exercised in drawing causal references from the results represented.

Data on many demographic variables were collected in the present study and the relationship between these variables and the key smoking, nutrition and sexual health variables, while having been analysed, have not always been presented in this report. Comparisons for individual demographic variables have only been presented where there are sufficient subjects within each stratum to be reasonably confident that the results were a reliable estimate. Respondents on various types of income benefits often differed greatly in their response to questions, but there were too few in these categories to make any detailed interpretation reliable.

Cluster analysis

So as not to lose important information about the demographic characteristics of the population, a cluster analysis has been used to derive a summary score for each person. This is a multivariate procedure for finding groups of respondents with similar characteristics in a file. No initial grouping was imposed on the data, but the object of the analysis was to see if individuals could be formed into any natural groups. Several types of variables can be used, including interval and dichotomous. The clusters formed can then be used in additional analyses. Cluster analysis was used, rather than principal component analysis, because the data were discretely, rather than continuously distributed.

The number of clusters was selected on the basis of a plot of the variance that remained within the cluster (R^2) against the number of clusters (varying from 1 to 9 clusters). Where the plot levels off, no further reduction of the within-cluster variance is achieved. The number of clusters corresponding with this point was chosen to be the best selected number of clusters. This gives the largest separation between the groups.

Although the cluster analysis provided a useful summary, caution should be exercised in the way the cluster analysis is interpreted. The internal consistency and logical groupings derived from the cluster analysis suggest, however, that the individual cluster score for each person does represent a reasonable proxy measure for the cluster of characteristics included in the analysis; that is to say there were no obvious inconsistencies in the way the cluster analysis grouped variables. The method has also been used by Peacock, Bland and Anderson (1995) and Huijbregts, Feskens and Kromhout (1995), and described by Armitage and Berry (1994).

Three new variables were computed using cluster analysis: one based on the demographic variables listed in Tables 2.4 to 2.15 (Table 2.1); the second based on the dietary questions to give an impression of the overall dietary behaviour (Table 2.2); and the third using the same demographic variables on the respondents to the sexual health questions (Table 2.3). The characteristics of the respondents in each cluster compared with the whole sample are described below. The variables are listed in the table in order of the size of the difference between the cluster and the sample mean. The variables which show the greatest difference from the sample mean are listed first, whilst those showing least variation are listed last.

Demographic clusters
The greatest difference between the groups was achieved using four clusters. Cluster 1 represented younger single subjects in full-time education or with some qualifications; cluster 2 also represented younger subjects but highlighted those with no formal education, lower income (on benefits), no use of a car, and those who were more likely to be living in overcrowded conditions. Clusters 3 and 4 differentiated between older age groups on the basis of professional qualifications; cluster 3 highlighted those with professional qualifications and non-manual occupations, and cluster 4 highlighted those with no formal qualifications and manual occupations (or retired). No value judgement has been made about the cluster groups which were derived independently by the analysis.

Table 2.1. Characteristics of respondents in each demographic cluster

Demographic cluster	Characteristics
1. Young educated	Full-time education; aged 16–19 years; have qualifications; single; no children; aged 20–24 years; 3 or more adults in household.
2. Younger, low-income families	Receiving income support; single parent; living in rented accommodation; receiving housing benefit; do not have use of a car; living in overcrowded conditions; looking after family/home – not employed; unemployed; no formal qualifications; manual occupation; aged 25–34 years.
3. Middle-aged educated	Have qualifications; two adults with children; have use of a car; employed; own property/have mortgage; non-manual occupation; aged 35–44 years.
4. Older, less educated	No formal qualifications; aged 65–74 years; retired couple; aged 55–64 years; retired single person; manual occupation

Dietary cluster

The greatest difference between the groups was achieved with two clusters. These clusters have been referred to as 'more' or 'less' healthy dietary clusters. Foods are listed in order of the magnitude of the difference between clusters. The more healthy cluster highlighted those respondents eating more wholemeal bread, using vegetable oils and low-fat spreads, whereas the less healthy cluster highlighted those using white bread and more whole milk.

Table 2.2. Characteristics of respondents in dietary clusters

Dietary cluster	Characteristics
1. More healthy	More wholemeal and brown bread; more likely to fry with vegetable oils and to use polyunsaturated margarines or low-fat spreads on bread; more skimmed milk; more likely to use polyunsaturated fats for cooking; more fruit; more fish.
2. Less healthy	More white bread; more whole milk; more likely to fry in lard; more fried foods; more likely to use butter or ordinary margarine on bread; more likely to use ordinary margarines for cooking; more burgers and sausages; more bacon, meat pies and processed meat.

Cluster analysis for the sexual health questionnaire

A separate cluster analysis was carried out for respondents who completed the sexual health questionnaire using the same demographic variables which were used for the demographic clusters. It was necessary to carry out a separate analysis as the age range and numbers of respondents differed from those completing the main questionnaire.

The greatest difference between the groups was achieved with two clusters which are referred to as cluster A and cluster B. The demographic variables which differed between the clusters are shown below.

Table 2.3. Characteristics of respondents in sexual health demographic clusters

Sexual health demographic cluster	Characteristics
1. Cluster A (worse off)	More likely to live in rented accommodation; receive income support; live in overcrowded conditions; receive housing benefit; to be a single parent; to be a manual worker.
2. Cluster B (better off)	More likely to have use of a car; to be employed.

Demographic characteristics of the respondents

Data from the Health and Lifestyle Survey 1993 have been compared with the Health Survey for England for 1991, 1992 and 1993 (a survey carried out by the Social Survey Division of OPCS on behalf of the Department of Health, which was designed to monitor trends in the nation's health) and the 1991 Census. Both weighted and unweighted figures are presented.

Weighting the data altered the relative proportions of men and women in the study (Table 2.4). For the weighted data there was the same proportion of men and women. Compared with the Health Survey for England and the 1991 Census there were relatively fewer women in the weighted data from the present survey. The unweighted proportion of women (58%) in the Health and Lifestyle Survey 1993 was slightly greater than either the Health Survey for England (54%) or the 1991 Census (52%).

Table 2.4. Percentage of men and women responding in the present study compared with the Health Survey for England 1993 and 1991 Census

	Men (%)	Women (%)
Health and Lifestyle Survey 1993 (n = 5 553)	50 (42)[1]	50 (58)[1]
Health Survey for England 1993 (n = 15 309)	46	54
Census 1991 (n = 35 million)	48	52

[1]Figures in brackets unweighted data

13

Table 2.5 shows the age structure for both men and women for all three surveys. The weighted data were similar to the 1991 Census population distribution. The respondents were selected to increase the 16–24 year age group and decrease the proportion of 55- to 74-year-olds and this was reflected when the Health and Lifestyle Survey 1993 was compared with the other surveys for the unweighted data. For the remaining age groups (25–44 years) the proportions were similar across the surveys. However, in men aged 45–54 there was a lower proportion than either the Health Survey for England 1993 (Bennett *et al.*, 1995) or the 1991 Census.

Table 2.5. Percentage distribution by respondents in the present study by gender compared with the Health Survey 1993 and 1991 Census

	Health and Lifestyle 1993 (%)	Health Survey 1993 (%)	Census 1991 (%)
Age (years)			
Men			
16–24	(22)[1] 17	15	18
25–34	(21) 22	21	21
35–44	(20) 19	19	19
45–54	(14) 17	18	16
55–64	(12) 14	15	14
65–74	(11) 11	13	11
n	(2 334) 2 754	7 228	18 million
Women			
16–24	(22)[1] 16	14	17
25–34	(23) 22	22	21
35–44	(18) 18	20	19
45–54	(16) 17	18	16
55–64	(11) 16	11	13
55–74	(10) 12	13	13
n	(3 219) 2 799	8 081	18 million

[1] Figures in brackets unweighted data

Table 2.6 shows the regional breakdown of the sample which was similar to both the Health Survey for England 1993 and the 1991 Census, although Anglia and Oxford was slightly overrepresented as a proportion of the total sample in the 1993 survey population. There was little difference between the weighted and unweighted data in the present survey.

Table 2.6. Percentage of respondents broken down by region in the present study compared with the Health Survey 1993 and 1991 Census

	Health and Lifestyle 1993 (%)	Health Survey 1993 (%)	Census 1991 (%)
Anglia & Oxford	(12)[1] 12	10	9
Northern & Yorks	(14) 14	15	14
Trent	(10) 10	10	10
North Thames	(13) 13	14	13
South Thames	(15) 14	15	14
South & West	(13) 13	13	13
West Midlands	(10) 11	9	11
North West	(14) 13	14	13
n	(5 553) 5 553	15 309	35 million

[1]Figures in brackets weighted data

Socioeconomic group of the respondent was used in preference to socioeconomic group of the head of household as around 20% of respondents had missing data for the head of household where it was not the respondent. Data were combined into non-manual and manual occupation groups (non-manual – professional, employers/managers, intermediate and junior non-manual; manual – skilled manual and own account non-professional, semi-skilled and unskilled manual) (Table 2.7). A higher proportion of women than men were defined as being in non-manual occupations.

Table 2.7. Percentage distribution of occupation group of the respondents in the present study by gender

	Men (%)	Women (%)
Non-manual	(45)[1] 45	(59)[1] 59
Manual	(50) 51	(33) 34
Never worked	(6) 4	(8) 7
n[2]	(2 260) 2 673	(3 150) 2 742

[1]Figures in brackets unweighted data
[2]Missing data for 3% men and 2% women

There were few differences in the distribution of marital status between the Health and Lifestyle Survey 1993 and the Health Survey for England 1992 (Breeze *et al.*, 1994) even after weighting the data (Table 2.8). Weighting the data reduced the proportion of respondents in the single and increased the proportion of respondents in the married categories.

Table 2.8. Percentage distribution of marital status of respondents in the present study by gender compared with the Health Survey 1992

	Men (%)		Women (%)	
	Health and Lifestyle Survey 1993	Health Survey 1992	Health and Lifestyle Survey 1993	Health Survey 1992
Married/cohabiting	(57)[1] 67	70	(58)[1] 69	66
Single	(34) 28	23	(24) 18	18
Separated/divorced	(6) 3	5	(10) 7	9
Widowed	(3) 2	2	(7) 6	8
n	(2 332) 2 753[2]	3 119	(3 215) 2 795[2]	3 517

[1]Figures in brackets unweighted data
[2]Missing data 0.1% for men and women

Table 2.9 summarises the work status of respondents in the survey in comparison with the Health Survey for England 1991 (White *et al.*, 1993). Inactive included retired respondents, those in full-time education, and those looking after the home. Similar results were observed for both surveys although more men in the present survey were employed than in the Health Survey. Women were most likely to be defined as inactive, presumably including those doing unpaid domestic work at home.

Table 2.9. Percentage distribution of work status of respondents in the present study by gender compared with the Health Survey 1991

	Men (%)		Women (%)	
	Health and Lifestyle Survey 1993	Health Survey 1991	Health and Lifestyle Survey 1993	Health Survey 1991
Employed	(62)[1] 64	59	(49)[1] 50	49
Unemployed	(11) 10	9	(4) 3	3
Inactive	(27) 26	28	(48) 47	48
n	(2 286) 2700[2]	7 228	(3 180) 2 767[2]	8 081

[1]Figures in brackets unweighted data
[2]Missing data 2% for men and 1% for women

The distribution of respondents' highest educational level in comparison with the Health Survey of England 1992 is summarised in Table 2.10. The present survey had a higher proportion with A levels or higher and other qualifications, and a lower proportion with no formal qualifications than the Health Survey. The 1993 General Household Survey (Foster *et al.*, 1995) showed that 31% of men and women combined had A level or higher qualifications.

Table 2.10. Percentage distribution of highest education level achieved by respondents in the present study by gender compared with the Health Survey 1992

	Men (%)		Women (%)	
	Health and Lifestyle Survey 1993	Health Survey 1992	Health and Lifestyle Survey 1993	Health Survey 1992
A levels or higher	(38)[1] 37	33	(27)[1] 26	23
Other (e.g. O levels)	(37) 37	34	(44) 41	38
No formal qualifications	(25) 26	31	(30) 33	39
n	(2 316) 2 734[2]	2 963	(3 201) 2 787[2]	3 340

[1]Figures in brackets unweighted data
[2]Missing data 1% for men and < 1% for women

Respondents were asked what type of accommodation they were currently living in. Responses were simplified into two broad categories of owner/occupier and rented (Table 2.11). The present survey showed a higher proportion in the owner/occupier category than the 1992 Health Survey. Around a quarter of the sample lived in rented accommodation; this was either rented from the council, housing association or privately rented.

Table 2.11. Percentage distribution of housing tenure of respondents in the present study by gender compared with the Health Survey 1992

	Men (%)		Women (%)	
	Health and Lifestyle Survey 1993	Health Survey 1992	Health and Lifestyle Survey 1993	Health Survey 1992
Own/being bought	(76)[1] 78	72	(72)[1] 76	71
Rent	(24) 22	28	(28) 24	29
n	(2 289) 2 704[2]	3 105	(3 149) 2 736[2]	3 509

[1]Figures in brackets unweighted data
[2]Missing data 2% for men and 2% for women

The bedroom standard was used to estimate housing occupation density by allocating a standard number of bedrooms to each household taking into account the age, gender, and marital status of members of the household and also the relation of members of the household to one another. A separate bedroom was allocated to each married couple, each adult aged 21 years or over, each pair of adolescents aged 10–20 years of the same gender, and each pair of children under 10 years of age. Unpaired persons aged 10–20 years may be paired with children under the age of 10 years. This figure was then compared with the actual number of bedrooms. Relatively few respondents lived in a household which did not meet the bedroom standard (Table 2.12).

Table 2.12. Percentage distribution of bedroom standard of respondents in the present study by gender

	Men (%)	Women (%)
Below standard	(4)[1] 4	(3)[1] 4
Meets standard	(27) 27	(28) 26
Above standard	(70) 69	(69) 71
n[2]	(2 315) 2 731	(3 181) 2 760

[1] Figures in brackets unweighted data
[2] Missing data for 1% men and 1% women

Table 2.13 summarises the distribution of household type by gender. The largest group of respondents were from households with three or more adults, followed by households with two adults and two children under 16 years of age. Weighting reduced the relative proportion of single persons compared with the unweighted responses. Very few men (1%) were single adults with children under 16 years compared with women (4%); we have referred to this group of single adults with children as single parents (mostly mothers) in the analyses.

Table 2.13. Percentage distribution of household type of respondents in the present study by gender

	Men (%)	Women (%)
Single	(13)[1] 7	(10)[1] 6
Single retired	(4) 3	(5) 4
Couple	(17) 18	(18) 19
Couple retired	(10) 11	(9) 12
3 or more adults	(21) 26	(15) 21
Single adult with children under 16 years	(1) 1	(9) 4
2 adults with children under 16 years	(24) 24	(25) 21
3 or more adults with children under 16 years	(10) 11	(9) 11
n[2]	(2 306) 2 729	(3 189) 2 774

[1] Figures in brackets unweighted data
[2] Missing data for 1% men and 1% women

Over 70% of men and women respondents stated that they had access to a car (Table 2.14). In the General Household Survey (Foster *et al.*, 1995) about 68% of respondents belonged to a household with a car.

Table 2.14. Percentage of respondents that own or have use of a car or van by gender

	Men (%)	Women (%)
Yes	(76)[1] 79	(71)[1] 76
n[2]	(2 331) 2 751	(3 214) 2 794

[1] Figures in brackets unweighted data
[2] Missing data for < 1% men and 1% women

Respondents were asked if they were receiving various benefits; the proportions receiving the main types of benefit are summarised in Table 2.15. Income support was the benefit most widely received by the sample; 7% of women were receiving housing benefit (weighted sample). Very few families received family credit or unemployment benefit. Given the current rate of unemployment (in 1993 – men 9%; women 5% – Foster *et al.*, 1995), the figures in the present study appear rather low.

Table 2.15. Percentage of respondents receiving various benefits by gender

	Men (%)	Women (%)
Income support	(9)[1] 8	(14)[1] 10
Unemployment benefit	(4) 4	(2) 3
Housing benefit	(5) 4	(9) 7
Family credit	(1) 1	(2) 2
n[2]	(2 334) 2 754	(3 219) 2 799

[1] Figures in brackets unweighted data
[2] No missing data

Table 2.16 presents the proportion of respondents in each demographic cluster. Cluster 2 had the smallest number of respondents and cluster 3 the greatest.

The division of respondents between the demographic clusters for the sexual health questionnaire is presented in Table 2.17. Three-quarters of respondents were included in cluster B.

Table 2.16. Percentage distribution of respondents by demographic cluster

Demographic cluster		%
1. Young educated	(29)[1]	24
2. Younger, low-income families	(13)	9
3. Middle-aged educated	(34)	38
4. Older, less educated	(25)	29
n[2]	(5 127)	5 135

[1] Figures in brackets unweighted data
[2] Missing data 8%

Table 2.17. Percentage distribution of respondents by sexual health demographic cluster

Sexual health demographic cluster		%
A Worse off	(29)[1]	24
B Better off	(71)	76
n[2]	(3 474)	3 475

[1] Figures in brackets unweighted data
[2] Missing data 6%

Appendix: The Kish grid

The Kish grid is a method for selecting the unit to investigate where there is more than one eligible unit at the address or household that should be interviewed (Kish, 1965; Moser and Kalton, 1979). In order to carry out the selection procedure the interviewer lists all eligible persons (in this case adults over 16 years of age) or all eligible households at the address; a number is then allocated to each person or household at the address. Eligible persons are listed in descending order of age, males followed by females. The persons are then numbered serially and the interviewer makes the selection by referring to the two lines of figures printed on the questionnaire.

References

Armitage, P and Berry, G (1994). *Statistical methods in medical research*. 3rd edn. Oxford: Blackwell Scientific.

Bennett, N, Dodd, T, Flatley, J, Freeth, S and Bolling, K (1995). *Health survey for England 1993*. London: HMSO.

Breeze, E, Maidment, A, Bennett, N, Flatley, J and Carey, S (1994). *Health survey for England 1992*. London: HMSO.

Foster, K, Jackson, B, Thomas, M, Hunter, P and Bennett, N (1995). *General household survey 1993*. London: HMSO.

Huijbregts, P P C W, Feskens, E J M and Kromhout, D (1995). Dietary patterns and cardiovascular risk factors in elderly men: the Zutphen Elderly Study. *International Journal of Epidemiology* **24**:313–20.

Kish, L (1965). *Survey sampling*. New York: Wiley.

Moser, C and Kalton, G (1979). *Survey methods in social investigation*. London: Heinemann Educational.

Peacock, J L, Bland, J M and Anderson, H R (1995). Preterm delivery: effects of socio-economic factors, psychological stress, smoking, alcohol, and caffeine. *British Medical Journal* **311**:5316.

Roe, L, Strong, C, Whiteside, C, Neil, A and Mant, D (1994). Dietary intervention in primary care: validity of the DINE method for dietary assessment. *Family Practice* **11**:375–81.

White, A, Nicolas, G, Foster, K, Browne, F and Carey, S (1993). *Health survey for England 1991*. London: HMSO.

3. Smoking

Introduction

This chapter summarises the main results from the analysis of the smoking data. The analysis has been divided into four sections: profile of smokers; smoking cessation; social issues; and health issues. The summaries and discussion draw out the main findings from the analysis. The objective of the analysis presented here has been to explore the important interactions in an attempt to get beyond a simple description of the data.

Profile of smokers

This section is presented in two parts: smoking status of respondents; and among smokers, levels of consumption.

- The overall prevalence of smoking appears to be declining for men but not for women; this survey reports rates of 29% (men) and 27% (women).
- Smoking rates are highest for:
  - women aged 20–24 (40%)
  - men aged 25–34 (37%)
  - separated or divorced women (44%)
  - men and women cohabiting (42%; 41%)
  - men and women with no formal qualifications (38%; 30%)
  - men and women in manual occupations (37%; 34%).
- Around half of all current smokers live in rented accommodation, are on income support or are unemployed.
- Over half of current smokers live in households with at least one other smoker.
- Over half of single mothers smoke.
- Over half of people living in younger, low-income families are smokers.
- Heavy smokers (20+ a day) are more likely to be men, manual workers, living in the North of England, or living in younger low-income families.

Smoking status of respondents

Table 3.1 presents the smoking status of respondents in the study. Respondents have been subdivided into those that are occasional or regular smokers, current or ex-smokers. This has been done because some other studies have only presented data on current regular smokers and presenting the subdivision allowed for comparison of prevalence rates with these studies. In comparison with the 1992 Health and Lifestyle Survey the overall prevalence of current smoking appears to have declined from 32% to 29% for men, but has remained unchanged for women at 27% in both surveys. Smoking prevalence in the present study was similar to that reported from the General Household Survey (Thomas *et al.*, 1994). The Health Survey for England conducted in 1993 (Bennett *et al.*, 1995) reported rates of current regular smokers of 28% for men and 26% for women, slightly below that reported in the present survey.

Table 3.1 Percentage distribution of smoking status of respondents by gender[1]

	Men (%)	Women (%)[2]
Total current smokers	**29**	**27**
Occasional cigarette smokers	3	2
Regular smokers	27	25 *
Total ex-smokers	**43**	**34**
Ex-occasional cigarette smokers	16	15 *
Ex-regular cigarette smokers	27	19
Never smoked cigarettes	**28**	**39**
Base:[3]	2 703	2 777

[1]Q173 SP derived from Q173/Q174/Q176/Q181. Have you ever smoked/do you smoke cigarettes at all nowadays/smoke regularly?
[2]Chi-squared test for all differences between men and women were statistically significant (p < 0.05) unless marked *
[3]Missing 2% men and 1% women

The higher percentage of men (43%) compared with women (34%) who said they were ex-smokers may be because some of the men are pipe and cigar smokers. Other surveys have shown that approximately 6% of males smoke cigars or pipes (Jarvis and Jackson, 1988). Women (39%) were more likely to report never regularly smoking cigarettes than men (28%). Unless otherwise specified smoking and smokers always refers to cigarettes.

When current smokers were broken down by age and gender the prevalence of cigarette smoking was highest in the 20–24 year age range for women and in the 25–34 year age range for men and lowest in the 55–74 year age ranges

(Figure 3.1). A higher proportion of women (40%) than men (34%) in the 20–24 year age range said they were current smokers; in all other age groups there were more men than women who smoked. There was a general decrease in the prevalence of cigarette smoking with age from 25–34 to 65–74 years. The trend with age was statistically significant for both men and women. The Health and Lifestyle Survey 1992 (HEA and MORI, 1995) showed that smoking prevalence was similar across all ages up to the age of 55 years after which it declined. The Health Survey for England 1993 showed that the smoking prevalence was higher in the younger than the older age groups. The Health Survey for England 1993 (Bennett *et al.*, 1995) also showed that trends for smoking behaviour during 1991, 1992, 1993 for men and women by age appear to be decreasing.

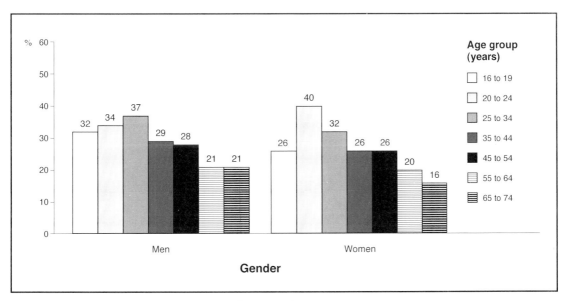

Mantel–Haenszel test for trend with age p < 0.05 for men and women

Fig. 3.1. Percentage distribution of cigarette smokers by age group by gender

The prevalence of smoking was broken down by the respondents' marital status (Figure 3.2). The highest smoking prevalence was observed for separated or divorced women (44%). A higher percentage of both men and women living with a partner (42% men and 41% women) reported that they were smokers compared to married people (25% men and 22% women). The differences between marital status groups were significantly different for married men versus single, cohabiting, separated/divorced and widowed; and for women all were significant except between married or single and widowed, and between separated or divorced and cohabiting. Thomas *et al.* (1994) also found that smoking levels were highest among the widowed, divorced or separated.

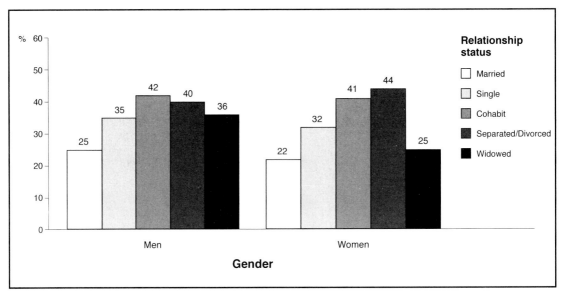

Chi-squared test for differences between marital status groups p < 0.05 for:
Men – married versus single, cohabit, separated/divorced and widowed
Women – all except single/married versus widowed; cohabit versus separated/divorced

Fig. 3.2. Percentage distribution of cigarette smokers by marital status by gender

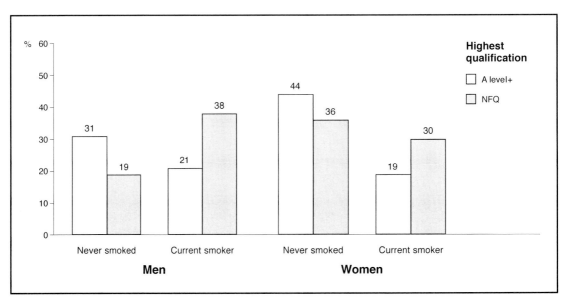

Chi-squared test for differences between qualification levels p < 0.05 for all
NFQ: no formal qualifications

Fig. 3.3. Percentage of cigarette smokers and never smokers by highest education qualification by gender

Subjects' highest educational achievement was subdivided into broad groups and Figure 3.3 presents the proportion of current and never smokers for those with an educational level of A level or above compared with those with no formal qualifications.

For men and women the proportion who said that they have never smoked was higher for respondents with A level or above than for those respondents with no formal qualifications (31% compared with 19% for men and 44% compared with 36% for women). For both men and women, respondents with no formal qualifications were more likely to smoke than those with A level or above qualifications (men – 38% compared with 21%; women – 30% compared with 19%).

The proportion of respondents who smoke was broken down by the type of work they reported (Figure 3.4). The proportion of manual workers who said that they smoked was higher than that for non-manual workers for both men and women. These differences were statistically significant for both men and women. Marsh and McKay (1994) found that smoking has halved among the better-off families in Britain but those on low incomes have continued to smoke at the same high rates as in the 1970s. The differences reported in the present study were similar to those reported in the 1992 Health and Lifestyle Survey.

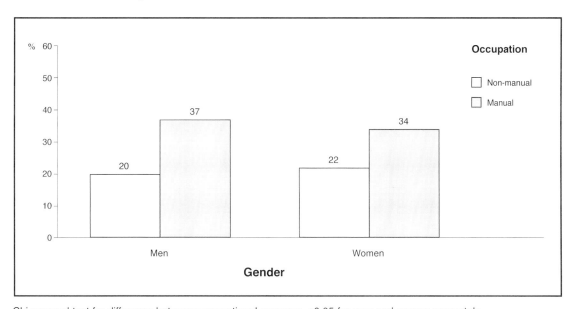

Chi-squared test for difference between occupational groups p < 0.05 for men and women separately

Fig. 3.4. Percentage of cigarette smokers by occupational group by gender

Smoking status (either current smoker or never smoked) was broken down by whether subjects lived in rented accommodation, were on income support and whether they were unemployed (Figure 3.5). A higher proportion of both

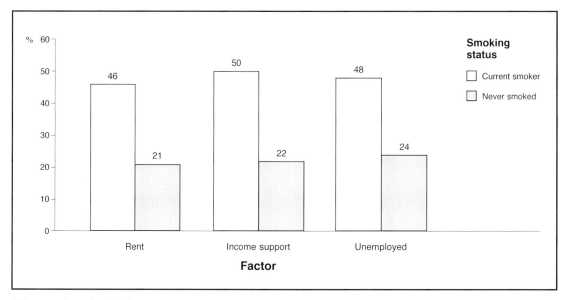

Chi-squared test for all differences between current smoker and never smoked p < 0.05

(i) Men

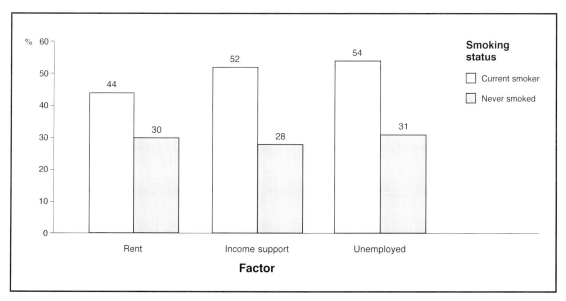

Chi-squared test for all differences between current smoker and never smoked p < 0.05 for all

(ii) Women

Fig. 3.5. Percentage of current smoker and never smoked by renting home, receiving income support and unemployment by gender

men and women who lived in rented accommodation or were on income support or were unemployed were smokers. The Health and Lifestyle Survey 1992 found that among individuals in rented accommodation, more than 40% were smokers. Marsh and McKay (1994) found that smoking was highest among council tenants receiving means-tested benefits. The Health and Lifestyle Survey 1992 also showed that just under half (46%) of people who were unemployed smoked, compared with 29% of those working and 36% of those economically inactive.

Fifty-five per cent of single mothers were current smokers. Cardozo *et al.* (1982) found that lone mothers appeared to be more likely to smoke, and smoke more heavily, than married or cohabiting mothers. Blackburn and Graham (1992) suggested that women may have found it easier to stop smoking and maintain smoking cessation if some of the material stresses associated with caring for children were relieved.

Figure 3.6 shows the percentage of respondents with smokers in their household broken down by smoking status. Fifty-seven per cent of men and 58% of women who reported they were current smokers lived in a household with at least one other smoker. This compared with 22% of men and 31% of women who were ex-smokers and 23% of men and 26% of women who had never smoked. The differences between smoking category by gender were statistically significant for current smokers with ex-smokers or never smokers.

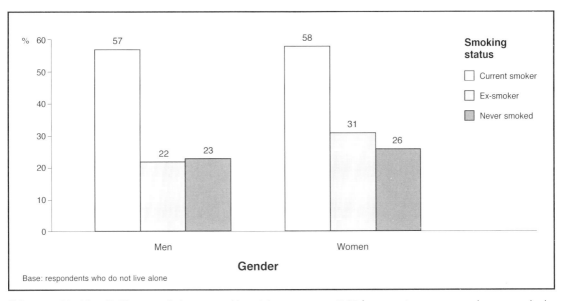

Chi-squared test for all differences between smoking status groups p < 0.05 for current versus ex- and never smoked

Fig. 3.6. Percentage of respondents with smokers in their household broken down by smoking status by gender

When the smoking status of respondents was broken down by the demographic cluster variable (Figure 3.7), 57% of respondents in younger, low-income families (cluster 2) reported that they smoked compared with 31% in the young, educated (cluster 1), 20% in the middle-aged, educated (cluster 3) and 27% in the older, less-educated (cluster 4).

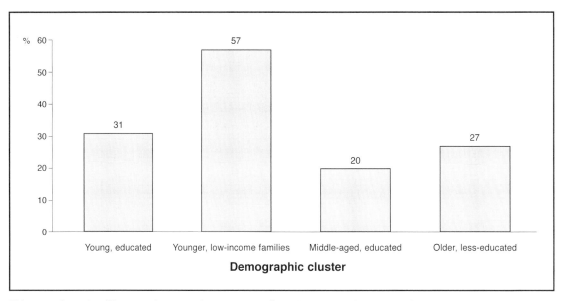

Chi-squared test for differences between cluster groups all p < 0.05 except for young, educated versus older, less-educated

Fig. 3.7. Percentage of cigarette smokers by demographic cluster group

When the smoking status of respondents was broken down by region there was no difference between the North and South in the prevalence of smoking for men (29% in each) but there was for women (North 29%; South 25%). Among men, but not women, there were more ex-smokers (men 45% compared with 41%) and fewer never smokers (26% compared with 30%), in the South compared with the North.

Cigarette consumption

Current regular smokers were asked about how many cigarettes they usually smoked on weekdays and at weekends; responses have been grouped into four broad categories (Table 3.2). Men were more likely than women to report smoking 40 or more cigarettes per day. Women were more likely than men to report smoking between 10 and 19 cigarettes a day. The difference between men and women was statistically significant. A similar proportion of men and women reported smoking between 1 and 9 cigarettes a day. Both men and women smoked more at the weekend than during the week. Thirty per cent of women in the Health Survey for England 1993 reported smoking less than

10 cigarettes a day compared with 22% in the Health and Lifestyle Survey 1992.

The Health and Lifestyle Survey 1992 found that the overall average daily cigarette consumption of regular smokers was 17; the number for the 1993 Health and Lifestyle Survey was 16. The present survey also found that women smoked fewer cigarettes per day than men at all ages (men = 17.6, women = 15.0) (Table 3.2).

Table 3.2. Percentage distribution of the number of cigarettes per day on weekdays and weekends by gender[1]

Cigs/day	Men (%)			Women (%)[2]		
	Weekdays	Weekend	Overall	Weekdays	Weekend	Overall
1 to 9	20	16	20	21	16	22*
10 to 19	37	28	37	44	41	44
20 to 39	38	47	39	33	40	33
40 or more	4	9	4	2	3	1
Average number of cigarettes	16.6	20.2	17.6	14.4	16.4	15.0
Base:[3]			722			691

[1]Q183 About how many cigarettes a day do you usually smoke on weekdays?
Q184 About how many cigarettes a day do you usually smoke at weekends?
(Average = (weekdays x 5) + (weekend days x 2)/7)
[2]Chi-squared test for differences between men and women statistically significant ($p < 0.05$) unless marked *
[3]Base: current regular cigarette smokers

The number of cigarettes respondents smoked per day was broken down by age and by gender (Figure 3.8). Fewer young people (16–24 age range) smoke 20 or more cigarettes a day compared with people in the older age range. The trend by age was statistically significant for number of cigarettes smoked per day except for 1–9 cigarettes a day for men and 10–19 cigarettes a day for women. The Health and Lifestyle Survey 1992 also found that in both men and women, consumption was highest among those aged 35–44 years and was lowest among those aged 16–24 years and aged 65–74 years.

When the number of cigarettes respondents smoked per day was broken down by broad occupational groups, a higher proportion of men and women who reported smoking 20 or more cigarettes a day were in the manual group (Figures 3.9(i)/(ii)) compared with the non-manual group. The differences by occupational group were statistically significant for women who smoked 1–9 and 20+ cigarettes a day. A similar proportion of men and women in both the manual and non-manual groups reported smoking 10 to 19 cigarettes a day. The Health and Lifestyle Survey 1992 found that consumption was highest among the occupational group IV–V for both men and women (equivalent to manual occupation in the present study).

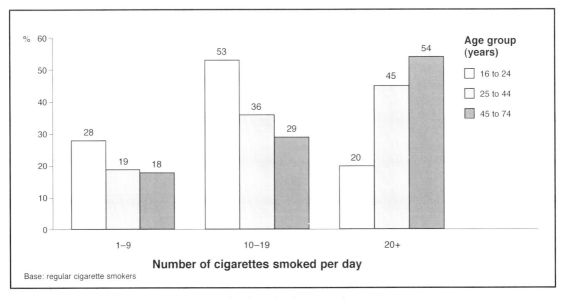

Mantel–Haenszel test for trend by age p < 0.05 for all levels of consumption

(i) Men

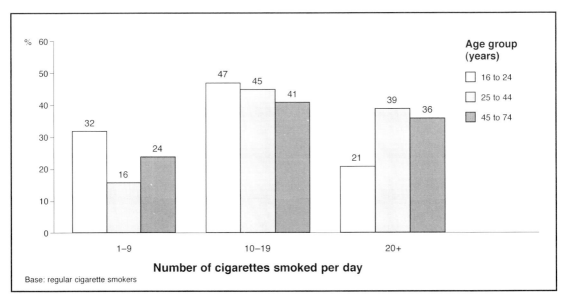

Mantel–Haenszel test for trend by age p < 0.05 for 20+ cigarettes only

(ii) Women

Fig. 3.8. Percentage distribution of daily cigarette consumption by age group by gender

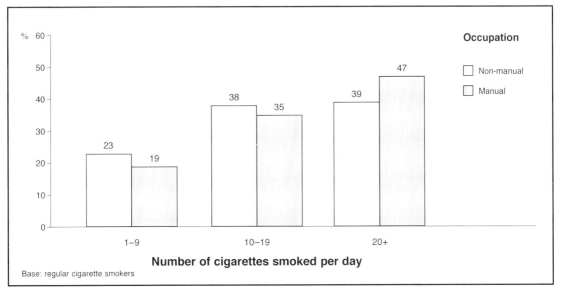

Chi-squared test for differences between occupational groups all p < 0.05

(i) Men

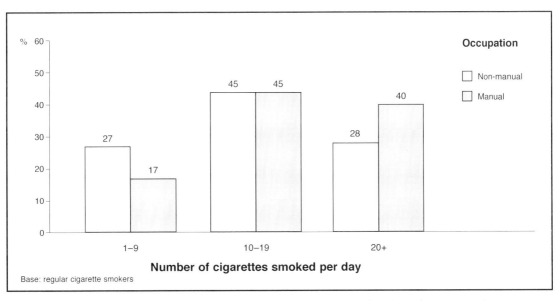

Chi-squared test for differences between occupational groups p < 0.05 except for 10–19 cigarettes per day

(ii) Women

Fig. 3.9. Percentage distribution of daily cigarette consumption by occupational group by gender

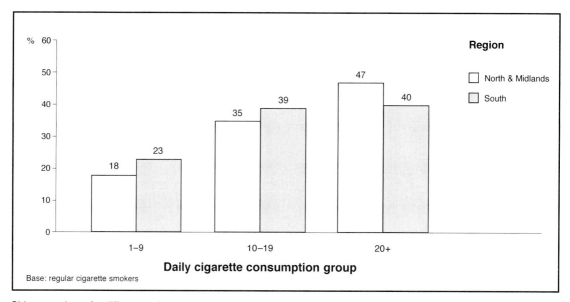

Chi-squared test for differences between regions p < 0.05 for 20+ cigarettes

(i) Men

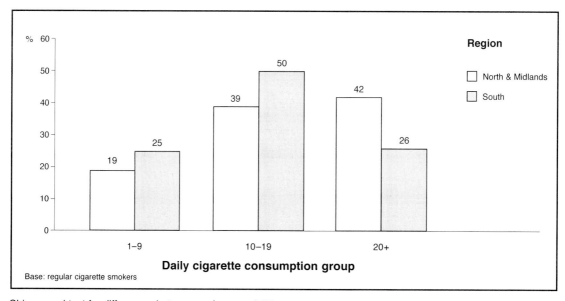

Chi-squared test for differences between regions p < 0.05

(ii) Women

Fig. 3.10. Percentage distribution of daily cigarette consumption groups by region by gender

When the number of cigarettes respondents smoked a day was broken down by region a higher proportion of men and women in the North compared with those in the South reported smoking 20 or more cigarettes a day (Figure 3.10(i)/(ii)). Regions were grouped this way for ease of presentation and also because there was relatively little variation between regions within the broad groupings presented here. This is similar to the Health and Lifestyle Survey 1992 that found in England, smokers in the North and Northwest reported a higher consumption than those in other parts of the country.

When the number of cigarettes respondents smoked per day was broken down by the demographic cluster, those in the young, educated (cluster 1) had the highest proportion of people who reported smoking 1–9 cigarettes a day and had the lowest proportion of 20 or more a day (Figure 3.13). Forty-six per cent of respondents in younger, low-income families (cluster 2) smoked 20 or more cigarettes per day.

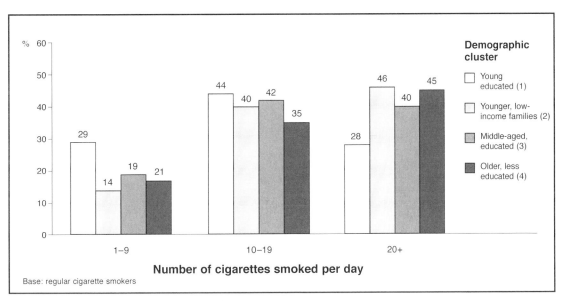

Chi-squared test for differences between clusters p < 0.05 for:
Young, educated with other clusters for 1–9, 20+ cigarettes smoked per day
Young, educated with older, less-educated for 10–19 cigarettes smoked per day

Fig. 3.11. Percentage distribution of daily cigarette consumption by demographic cluster group

Smoking cessation

This section explores the characteristics of current and ex-smokers with respect to patterns of onset and establishment of smoking habits and attempts to stop smoking.

- Women are increasingly starting to smoke at younger ages.

- Manual workers are more likely to start smoking before the age of 16 than non-manual workers.

- Over a quarter of respondents in younger, low-income families started to smoke before the age of 16.

- The older men and women were when they first tried cigarettes and when they started smoking regularly, the more likely they are to be able to stop.

- Most ex-smokers gave up between the ages of 25 and 34 years.

- Over half of current smokers have failed in attempts to stop smoking for 12 months.

- Occupational group has no effect on success or failure at cessation attempts for men. But more women in manual occupations fail in their attempts to stop than in non-manual occupations.

- Men and women who smoke less are more likely to succeed in giving up.

- Women living with a smoker and smokers in younger, low-income families are less likely to try to stop, and to be successful if they do.

Onset and establishment of smoking

Current regular smokers and ex-smokers were asked how old they were when they first tried smoking (Table 3.3). Forty-one per cent of men and

Table 3.3. Percentage distribution of the age smokers and ex-smokers first tried smoking by gender[1]

Age (years)	Men (%)		Women (%)[2]	
	Smokers	Ex-smokers	Smokers	Ex-smokers
Up to 11	14	5	14	4
11–13	27	20	22	15
14–15	30	31*	34	27
16+	30	44	29	53
Base:[3]	715	685	720	536

[1]Q175/Q180. How old were you when you first tried smoking?
[2]Chi-squared test for differences between men and women all statistically significant p < 0.05 unless marked *
[3]Base: current regular cigarette smokers and ex-regular cigarette smokers. Missing ≤ 1% men and women

20–25% of women current smokers first tried smoking under the age of 14 years. Women who were ex-smokers were more likely to have first tried smoking at an older age than current smokers (16+ years – ex-smokers 53%, smokers 44%). There were statistically significant differences between all age groups, except for 14- to 15-year-olds, and between men and women.

Around half of the respondents who have ever smoked reported starting to smoke regularly (one or more cigarettes per day) between the ages of 16 and 19 years (Table 3.4). Women were more likely than men to have started smoking after 20 years of age; ex-smokers were more likely to have started regular smoking at a later age than current smokers. Cox *et al.* (1987) found that the main ages for taking up smoking for both men and women were around 14–16 years old, and after the age of 20 very few people take up regular smoking. This survey shows that between 16% and 29% of men and women have taken up regular smoking after the age of 20 years.

Table 3.4. Percentage distribution of the age smokers and ex-smokers started to smoke regularly by gender[1]

Age (years)	Smokers (%)		Ex-smokers (%)[2]	
	Men	Women	Men	Women
Up to 11	2	<1	1	<1 *
11–13	9	6*	4	4 *
14–15	23	19	24	12
16–19	51	51*	55	55 *
20+	16	24	17	29
Base:[3]	716	683	720	534

[1]Q182/Q177. How old were you when you started to smoke cigarettes regularly?
[2]Chi-squared test for differences between men and women statistically significant $p < 0.05$ unless marked *
[3]Base: current regular cigarette smokers and ex-regular cigarette smokers. Missing ≤ 1% men and women

Figure 3.12 shows that there was little variation by the respondents' current age in the percentage of men who reported starting to smoke regularly before the age of 16 (range 15–19% across age groups). However, in women aged 16 to 19 years, the percentage who reported starting to smoke regularly before the age of 16 years was 17% compared with only 5% of the 65 to 74 years age group. The trend for starting to smoke at a younger age was statistically significant for women only. There may be effects of memory on reporting, sample selection due to ill health in older long-term smokers, marital status and other factors related to age suggesting a secular trend. However, as this is seen for women only, these data would suggest that there is an underlying tendency towards earlier commencement of smoking in women.

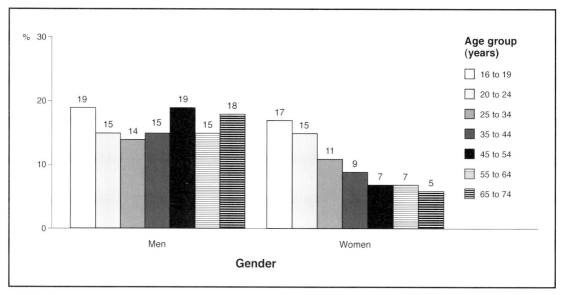

Mantel–Haenszel test for trend p < 0.05 for women only

Fig. 3.12. Percentage of respondents starting to smoke before the age of 16 years by current age by gender

A higher proportion of manual workers than non-manual workers, for both men and women, started smoking before the age of 16 years (Figure 3.13).

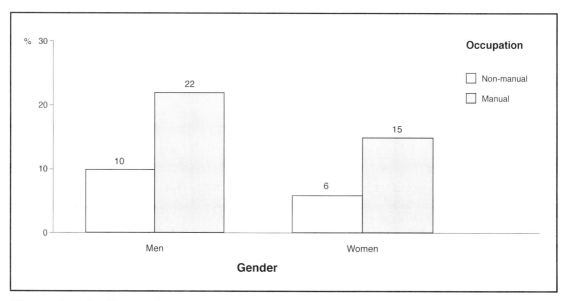

Chi-squared test for differences between occupational groups p < 0.05

Fig. 3.13. Percentage of respondents starting to smoke before the age of 16 years by occupational group by gender

Just over a quarter of respondents in demographic cluster 2 (younger low-income families) compared with 8% in cluster 3 (middle-aged, better educated) started to smoke before the age of 16 (Figure 3.14). The differences between clusters were all statistically significant.

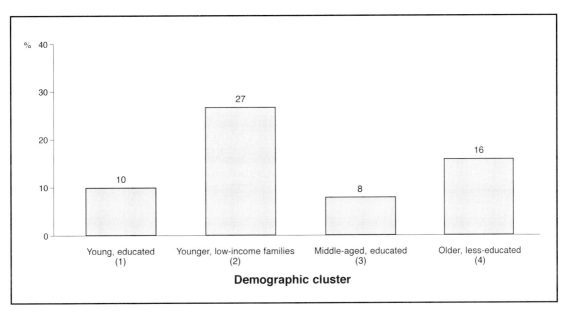

Chi-squared test for differences between clusters p < 0.05 for all

Fig. 3.14. Percentage of respondents starting to smoke before the age of 16 years by demographic cluster group

Influences on success and failure in stopping smoking

Ex-regular smokers were asked how long ago they stopped smoking cigarettes regularly (Table 3.5). Nearly a third of men and 24% of women had stopped smoking for at least 20 years; 37% of women had stopped in the last 5 years compared with 27% for men (these differences were statistically significant).

Age at stopping smoking was computed from respondents' current age and the answer to the question on how long ago they stopped smoking regularly (Figure 3.15). The highest proportion of both men and women reported giving up smoking between the ages of 25 and 34 years (32% for men; 30% for women). There were too few subjects in each age/gender group to allow further analysis.

Table 3.5. Percentage distribution of years since ex-smokers stopped regular smoking by gender[1]

	Men (%)	Women (%)[2]
Less than 1 year	8	11
Up to 5 years	19	26
Up to 10 years	10	13 *
Up to 15 years	18	15 *
Up to 20 years	13	11 *
20 or more years	32	24
Base:[3]	719	536

[1]Q179 How long ago did you stop smoking cigarettes regularly?
[2]Chi-squared test for differences between men and women statistically significant (p < 0.05) unless marked *
[3]Base: ex-regular smokers. Missing ≤ 1% men and women

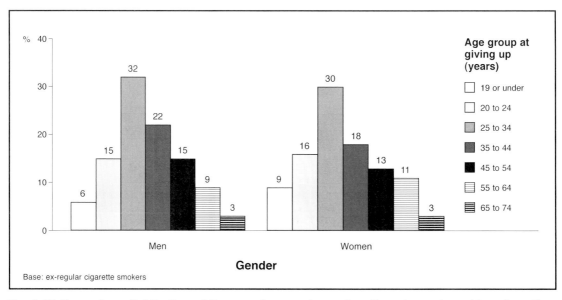

Fig. 3.15. Percentage distribution of the age of ex-smokers when they stopped smoking cigarettes regularly by gender

Figure 3.16 presents the proportion of current smokers who have tried to stop smoking for at least 12 months. For both men and women about a quarter of current smokers have never tried to stop smoking and 55–58% tried and failed. Under 20% of men and women reported that they had successfully stopped smoking for at least 12 months. There were no statistically significant differences between men and women in their responses to this question.

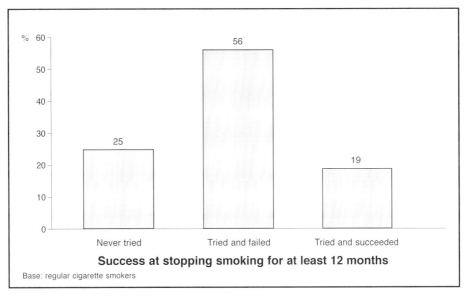

Fig. 3.16. Percentage distribution of success at stopping smoking for at least 12 months (genders combined)

This survey did not have any questions about smokers' desire to quit. The Health and Lifestyle Survey 1992 found that a large proportion of smokers expressed a wish to give up smoking (64% of male smokers and 65% of female smokers). The NOP Survey on Smoking Habits (Department of Health, 1994a) found that 61% of adults aged 16 years and over who reported being regular smokers wanted to stop smoking altogether. The Health and Lifestyle Survey 1992 found that 80% of smokers reported having made one or more attempts to give up smoking.

This survey did not provide data on how many times ex-smokers reported that they had tried to give up prior to succeeding. The Health and Lifestyle Survey 1992 found that more than 50% of respondents reported having succeeded at their first attempt.

The demographic characteristics of smokers who had successfully given up for more than 12 months compared with those that had not tried or who had tried but failed, were explored further. Figure 3.17 (i)/(ii) presents responses broken down by occupational group. For men there were no statistically significant differences in responses by occupational group. For women, a greater proportion of manual than non-manual workers reported they had tried and failed to stop smoking (64% compared with 46%) and fewer had been successful at stopping for 12 months (13% compared with 26%).

West (1995) reported that the widening gap between smoking rates in different socioeconomic groups was partly because smokers in more deprived sections of society are less likely to give up. Yet smokers in more

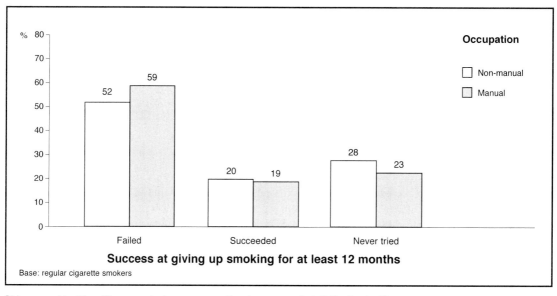

Chi-squared test for differences between occupational groups not statistically significant

(i) Men

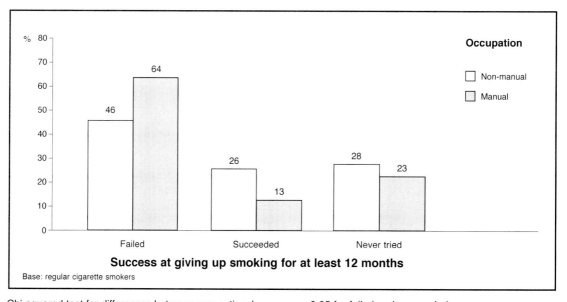

Chi-squared test for differences between occupational groups p < 0.05 for failed and succeeded

(ii) Women .

Fig. 3.17. Percentage distribution of success at stopping smoking for at least 12 months by occupational group

deprived socioeconomic groups are just as likely to express a desire to stop as more prosperous smokers. West (1995) proposed that the main social class difference was due to difficulty giving up once an attempt has been made, indicating a need to look at appropriate support for smokers in lower socioeconomic groups. Buck and Godfrey (1994) reported that intensive general practitioner advice or advice to buy nicotine gum or patches appeared to be more effective than a brief consultation. However, the effectiveness of such interventions depends heavily on the willingness of patients to spend either time in attending the GP surgery, or money in purchasing nicotine gum or patches.

To explore whether the intensity of cigarette smoking was associated with whether subjects reported to have successfully stopped smoking for at least a year, Figure 3.18 summarises the distribution of cigarettes smoked per day broken down by success at stopping smoking. Both men and women who smoked less reported a higher success rate for giving up. It is not possible to tell from these data whether the people who quit were 'lifetime' smokers of one to nine cigarettes a day, or whether they had cut down to this from a higher number of cigarettes per day and then given up. If so, there could be implications for the approach used by health professionals involved in smoking campaigns – to encourage people to cut down prior to giving up.

Respondents in demographic cluster 2 (younger, low-income families) were less likely to have tried and succeeded in giving up cigarettes than respondents in cluster 3 (middle-aged, educated) (12% compared with 26%). Marsh and McKay (1994) also found that half of the better-off young smokers gave up, and the poorer smokers found it more difficult.

Women who were successful at stopping smoking were less likely to live with a smoker (46%) than those who had tried and failed (58%) and those who had never tried (63%). These differences were statistically significant for women but no statistically significant differences were seen for men.

Subjects' success at stopping smoking was broken down by age at starting smoking (Figure 3.19(i)/(ii)). Both men and women who started smoking before the age of 16 years were more likely to have tried and failed to stop smoking than respondents who started at an older age. The older men and women were when they started smoking the more likely they were to have been able to stop smoking.

No data were obtained on factors precipitating relapse or the main advantages for giving up. The Health and Lifestyle Survey 1992 found that the most commonly reported factors for relapse were stress and willpower; for the main advantages of giving up the majority of smokers reported improvement to their current health (50%) and saving money (59%).

The present survey did not obtain data on reasons given by ex-smokers for having stopped smoking. The Health and Lifestyle Survey 1992 found that the most commonly reported reasons were those related to health. The Health

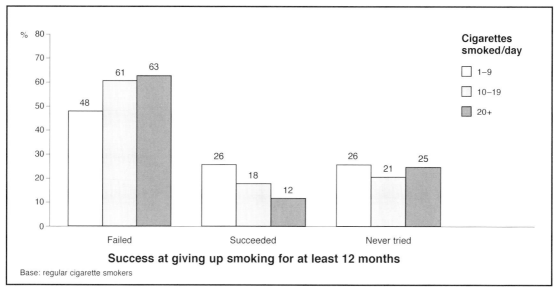

(Mantel–Haenszel test for trend with number of cigarettes p < 0.05 for failed and succeeded

(i) Men

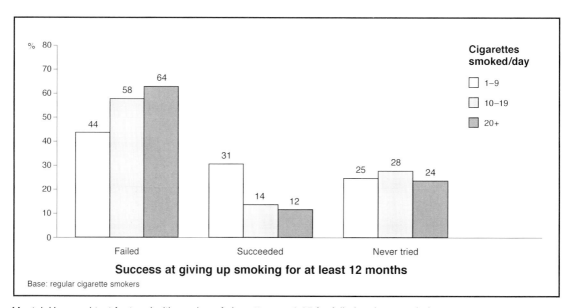

Mantel–Haenszel test for trend with number of cigarettes p < 0.05 for failed and succeeded

(ii) Women

Fig. 3.18. Percentage distribution of success at stopping smoking for at least 12 months by number of cigarettes smoked per day by gender

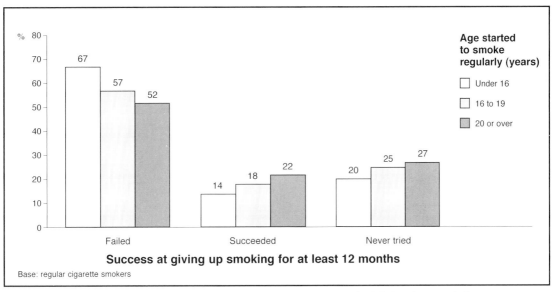

Mantel–Haenszel test for trend with age started to smoke regularly p < 0.05 for failed and succeeded

(i) Men

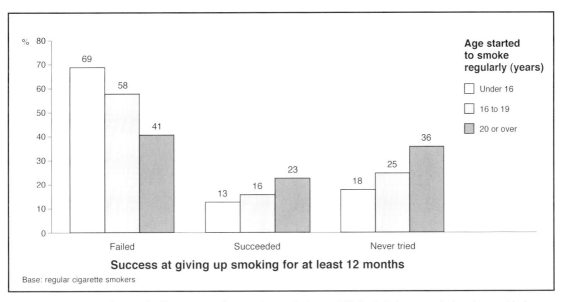

Mantel–Haenszel test for trend with age started to smoke regularly p < 0.05 for failed, succeeded and never tried

(ii) Women

Fig. 3.19. Percentage distribution of success at stopping smoking by age started to smoke regularly by gender

and Lifestyle Survey 1992 asked ex-smokers what methods they had used to give up smoking. The majority of both men and women said that they had not used any particular aid. Approximately 20% cited support from their family and friends. Advice from a doctor was reported by 4% of women and 9% of men. Aids from the chemist such as nicotine gum were reported by 6% of men and 5% of women. Telephone helplines were used very rarely, as were alternative therapies such as acupuncture and hypnosis.

Social issues

This section explores the rules respondents had about visitors smoking in their homes and how confident they felt about restricting smoking in their homes. For smokers it examines the situations in which they would not smoke and their attitudes to smoking near babies, young children and pregnant women, and to smoking in pregnancy.

- Smokers and non-smokers are generally permissive in their attitudes towards allowing visitors to smoke in their homes.

- Women, and older people feel less confident about asking visitors not to smoke.

- Half of current smokers feel they should not smoke in restaurants, younger smokers are less likely to agree with this.

- Not smoking near babies, children or pregnant women seems to be widely accepted. However there appears to be less acceptance of the need to stop smoking in pregnancy by older people, men, and women in manual occupations.

- Smokers in younger, low-income families and the older, less-educated group are more likely than others to ignore smoking bans in public places.

Rules about smoking

All respondents were shown cards with statements describing rules about visitors smoking in their home and asked which of these best described what happened when they had visitors in their home (Table 3.6). Two-thirds of all respondents (whether smokers or not) indicated that visitors were allowed to smoke in their home if they wished (women statistically significantly more so than men). Men were more likely than women (18% compared with 15%) to say that no visitors were allowed to smoke in their home.

When subjects' response to the question about visitors being allowed to smoke in their home was examined by smoking status (Figure 3.20) more current smokers (84% men and 89% women) reported allowing all visitors to smoke in their home than ex-smokers (59% men and 61% women) or those who have never smoked (48% men and 55% women). The differences were statistically significant between smoking status groups.

Table 3.6. Percentage distribution of respondents' rules about visitors smoking in respondents' homes by gender[1]

	Men (%)	Women (%)[2]
All visitors are allowed to smoke in my home if they wish	63	66 †
Some visitors are allowed to smoke in my home, others may not	10	9
No visitors are allowed to smoke in my home	18	15 †
We never have visitors who might want to smoke	7	7
We never have visitors	<1	<1
It depends	2	3
Don't know/no answer	1	1
Base:	2 754	2 799

[1]Q202 Which of these best describes what happens when you have visitors in your home?
[2]Chi-squared test for differences between men and women statistically significant (p < 0.05) if marked †

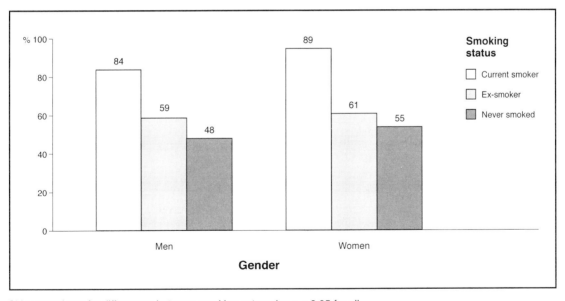

Chi-squared test for differences between smoking categories p < 0.05 for all

Fig. 3.20. Percentage of respondents indicating that all visitors are allowed to smoke in their home by respondents' smoking status by gender

Whether visitors were allowed to smoke in the respondents' home was examined by occupational group (Figure 3.21). A higher proportion of manual workers, for both men and women, reported that 'all visitors are allowed to smoke in my home if they wish'. The differences between occupational groups were statistically significant for both men and women. There was no difference across the age range or for marital status in respondents' attitudes about visitors smoking in the home.

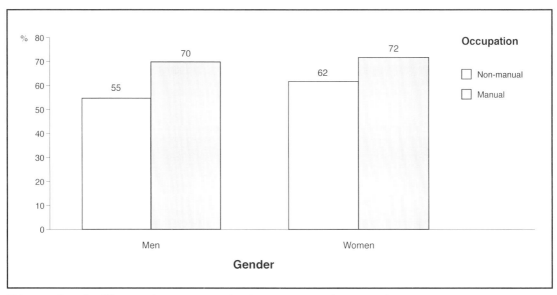

Chi-squared test for differences between occupational groups p < 0.05 for men and women

Fig. 3.21. Percentage of respondents indicating that all visitors are allowed to smoke in their home by respondents' occupational group by gender

When the likelihood of visitors being allowed to smoke was analysed by cluster group (Figure 3.22) a higher proportion of people in younger, low-income families (cluster 2) and the older, less-educated (cluster 4) said that they allowed visitors to smoke in their home than in clusters 1 and 3.

Those respondents who answered that all/some/no visitors were allowed to smoke in their home were then asked if they did not want visitors to smoke in their home, how confident would they feel about asking visitors not to smoke (Table 3.7). Men (59%) were statistically significantly more likely than women (43%) to feel very confident about asking visitors not to smoke; 31% of women and 15% of men were either not very, or not at all, confident about asking visitors not to smoke. Those respondents who did not feel confident about asking visitors not to smoke in their home were asked: Why would you not feel very or at all confident about asking visitors not to smoke in your home? Responses included: not up to me to decide who smokes here (10%), feel too embarrassed to ask (20%), don't want to offend people (34%), don't want to be unfriendly (20%) and I smoke myself (7%).

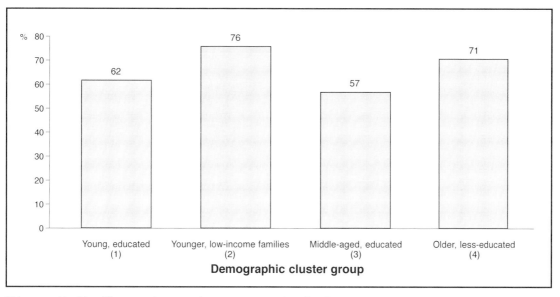

Chi-squared test for differences between cluster groups p < 0.05 for all

Fig. 3.22. Percentage of respondents indicating that all visitors are allowed to smoke in their home by demographic cluster group

Table 3.7. Percentage distribution of respondents   **confidence in**
asking visitors not to smoke in their home by gender[1]

	Men (%)	Women (%)[2]
Very confident	59	43
Fairly confident	20	22
Not very confident	10	21
Not at all confident	5	10
Don't know/no answer	6	4
Base:[3]	2489	2512

[1]Q204 If you did not want visitors to smoke in your home, how confident would you feel about asking them not to?
[2]Chi-squared test for differences between men and women statistically significant p < 0.05 for all
[3]Base: respondents who answered all/some/no visitors are allowed to smoke in my home

When subjects' confidence about asking visitors not to smoke in their homes was broken down by age (Figure 3.23) women reported feeling less confident than men across the age range. In general for both men and women, respondents in the older age groups were less confident about asking visitors not to smoke in their home than younger respondents. These trends by age were statistically significant for men and women. Further analysis showed little difference by smoking status and occupational group.

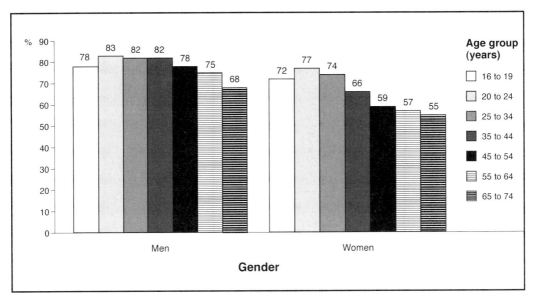

Mantel–Haenszel test for trend with age p < 0.05 for men and women separately

Fig. 3.23. Percentage in each age group who feel confident to ask visitors not to smoke in their homes by gender

Where smokers feel they should not smoke

Current smokers were shown a card and asked to indicate whether there were any situations where they felt they should not smoke (Table 3.8). Almost all respondents (91% of men and 93% of women) felt they should not smoke in doctors' surgeries and health centres. Only about half the respondents felt they should not smoke in restaurants or places where people were eating nearby. About three-quarters felt that they should not smoke when they were with others who were eating.

When respondents who felt that they should not smoke in restaurants were broken down by age group, more men aged 25–44 years (62%) felt that they should not smoke in restaurants than 16- to 24-year-olds (52%). More women aged 45–74 years (67%) felt they should not smoke in restaurants compared with 16- to 24-year-olds (53%) and 25- to 44-year-olds (53%).

The Health and Lifestyle Survey 1992 found that there was widespread support for smoking restrictions in many public places. Relatively few people said they would support a policy of allowing unrestricted smoking in any of the kinds of public places asked about. The only exception was pubs where a quarter of adults (25%) supported allowing smoking everywhere.

More people felt they shouldn't smoke near babies/young children than near pregnant women or during pregnancy. Further analysis of responses related to smoking near babies/young children showed no difference by age groups. Most men and women reported that they felt they should not smoke near babies/young children. However, only 62% of women reported that they felt they should not smoke in pregnancy. When smoking near pregnant women was analysed by age group for men and women, younger people were more likely to have reported that they felt they should not smoke near pregnant women than older people (men 16–19 years 65%; 65–74 years 46%; women 16–19 years 64%; 65–74 years 58%) although the trends across all age groups were not statistically significant for either men or women. When smoking during pregnancy was analysed by age group a higher proportion of young women reported that they felt they should not smoke during pregnancy (Figure 3.24). The trend by age was statistically significant.

Table 3.8. Percentage distribution of places/situations where smokers feel they should not smoke by gender[1]

	Men (%)	Women (%)[2]
Doctors' surgeries/health centres	91	93
Hospital waiting areas	86	88
Restaurants/places where people are eating nearby	59	58
The homes of people who do not smoke	77	81
Near babies/young children	75	80 †
Near pregnant women	57	53
On public transport	49	53
Other public places	22	29 †
When with others who are eating	72	78
Aeroplanes	32	34
Shops	60	68 †
Public toilets	20	36 †
In the street	7	35 †
All places where there is a smoking ban	78	81
During pregnancy	39	62 †
Other	2	<1 †
None	1	<1
Don't know/no answer	2	2
Base:[3]	794	735

[1] Q207 Are there any places or situations where you feel you should not smoke?
[2] Chi-squared test for differences between men and women statistically significant $p < 0.05$ if marked †
[3] Base: regular cigarette smokers

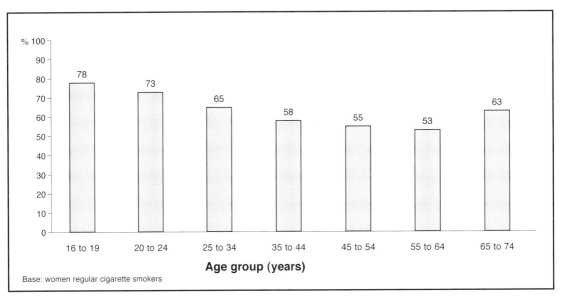

Mantel–Haenszel test for trend with age p < 0.05

Fig. 3.24. Percentage of women respondents who feel they shouldn't smoke during pregnancy by age group

Smoking near pregnant women/during pregnancy was examined by occupation group (Figure 3.25). A higher proportion of non-manual men and women felt that they should not smoke near pregnant women. More women than men felt women should not smoke during pregnancy. There was no difference between non-manual and manual groups for men, but more non-manual women thought they would not smoke during pregnancy.

Smoking near babies/young children, near pregnant women and during pregnancy was broken down by the demographic cluster (Figure 3.26) Overall the greater proportion in each cluster were more likely to feel they should not smoke near babies and young children than during pregnancy. Even within the middle-aged better-educated (cluster 3) only 50% of respondents felt they should not smoke during pregnancy, whereas 80% felt they should not smoke near babies/young children.

Respondents in clusters 2 and 4 (young, low-income families and older less-educated) were less likely to feel they should not smoke near any of the groups indicated.

Respondents in clusters 2 and 4 were also more likely to smoke where there was a smoking ban (Figure 3.27).

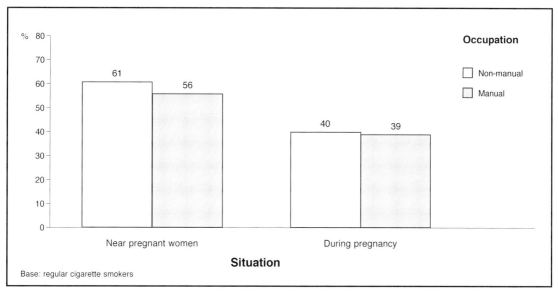

Chi-squared test for differences between occupational groups were not statistically significant

(i) Men

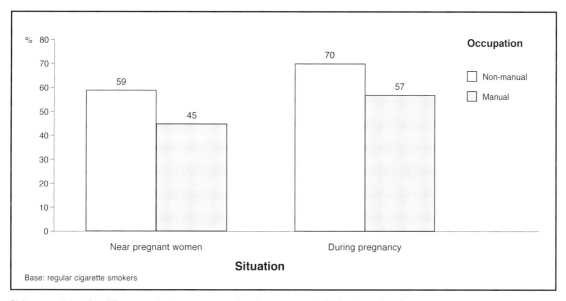

Chi-squared test for differences between occupational groups p < 0.05 for both situations

(ii) Women

Fig. 3.25. Percentage of respondents who feel they shouldn't smoke near pregnant women and during pregnancy by occupation

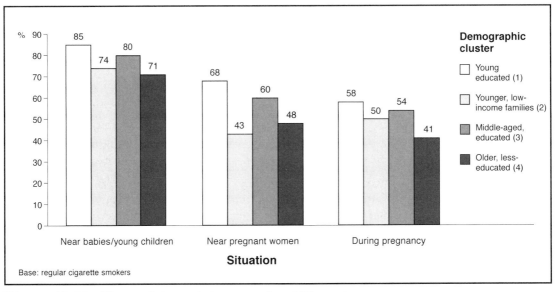

Chi-squared test for differences between cluster groups all p < 0.05 except
Near babies 1 v. 3, 2 v. 3, 2 v. 4; Near pregnant women 2 v. 4; During pregnancy 1 v. 2 and 3, 2 v. 3

Fig. 3.26. Percentage of respondents who feel they shouldn't smoke near babies/young children, near pregnant women and during pregnancy by demographic cluster group

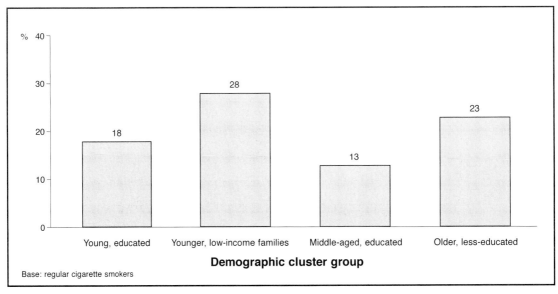

Chi-squared test for differences between cluster groups p < 0.05 for:
Young, educated versus younger, low-income, families; Younger, low-income, families versus middle-aged, educated; Middle-aged educated versus older, less-educated

Fig. 3.27. Percentage of each cluster group who felt they would smoke in places where there is a smoking ban

Health issues

This section explores smokers' perceptions of the effects of smoking on their own health, and that of their children, and of the effects on health of passive smoking in general.

- More younger than older smokers feel that their smoking was affecting their health. Nearly two-fifths of those smoking 20 or more a day felt that it had little or no effect on their health.

- Few of those acknowledging a health effect mentioned cancer or heart disease; breathlessness, cough and for men fitness, were more important. Heavy smokers were no more likely to be concerned about long-term health effects than lighter smokers.

- People who have never smoked are more likely to believe that passive smoking has a great deal of effect on other people's health than current smokers.

- Younger people are more likely to believe that passive smoking affects health than older people.

- Over one-third of parents (where there was a smoker in the household) thought the health of their children was not affected at all by their smoking.

- Of all parents who had children under 16, 57% of men and 43% of women felt that parental smoking made children more likely to smoke.

- Smoking parents appear not to recognise the impact of their smoking on the likelihood of their children smoking. Only 31% of men and 22% of women thought that their children would be more likely to smoke while 16% of men and 26% of women thought that their children would be less likely to smoke.

Smokers' perceptions of the effect of smoking on own health

Current smokers were asked how much, if at all, they would say their smoking affected their health (Table 3.9). The differences between men and women were not statistically significant. About half of men and women perceived smoking as having a great deal or a fair amount of effect on their health; about 20% of men and women thought smoking did not affect their health at all. The Health and Lifestyle Survey 1992 found that the large majority of smokers believed that their smoking was actually affecting their current health.

Table 3.9. Percentage distribution of smokers' perceptions of the extent of effect of smoking on their health by gender[1]

	Men (%)	Women (%)[2]
A great deal	22	22
A fair amount	28	28
Just a little	27	25
Not at all	19	21
Don't know/no answer	4	4
Base:[3]	794	735

[1]Q216 How much, if at all, would you say your smoking affects your health?
[2]Chi-squared test for differences not statistically significant
[3]Base: regular cigarette smokers

When smokers' perception of the extent of the effect of smoking on their health was analysed by age group (Figure 3.28(i)/(ii)) more younger smokers than older smokers perceived that smoking affected their health a great deal or a fair amount. The trend was statistically significant with age. Further analysis showed little difference in the perception of effects on health when broken down by marital status or occupational group.

Smokers' perceptions of the extent of the effect of smoking on their health were analysed by the number of cigarettes smoked per day (Figure 3.29(i)/(ii)). For both men and women there was a statistically significant trend towards increasing perception of the effect of smoking on health the more cigarettes smoked a day. However, 39% of men and 38% of women who smoked 20 or more cigarettes a day reported that smoking had little or no effect on their health. The Health and Lifestyle Survey 1992 found that the proportion of people who believed that smoking was adversely affecting their health was greater for heavier smokers.

Current smokers who answered that smoking affects their health a great deal/fair amount or just a little were asked in what ways they would say that smoking affected their health (Table 3.10). Just over 40% of men and women felt that smoking affected their breathlessness, 24% mentioned coughing and among men 19% said that it affected their fitness. Few men and women felt that smoking affected their risk of cancer (8% for women, 12% for men). 'Other' responses included the following: less appetite control; lung problems; food has less taste; colds are worse; affects the skin; cardiovascular problems; sore throats; problems in the future; tiredness/lethargy; stains teeth; calmer; causes bad breath and chest problems.

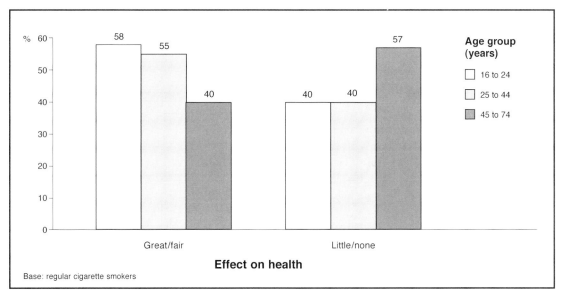

Mantel–Haenszel test for trend with age p < 0.05

(i) Men

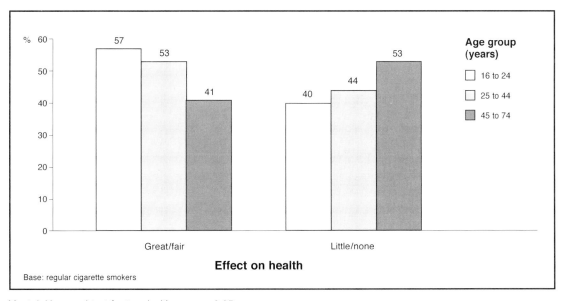

Mantel–Haenszel test for trend with age p < 0.05

(ii) Women

Fig. 3.28. Percentage distribution of smokers' perception of how smoking affects their health by age group by gender

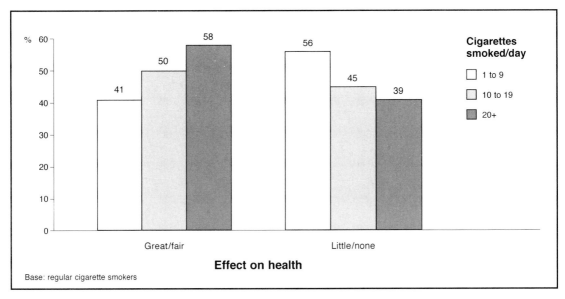

Mantel–Haenszel test for trend with number of cigarettes p < 0.05 for each

(i) Men

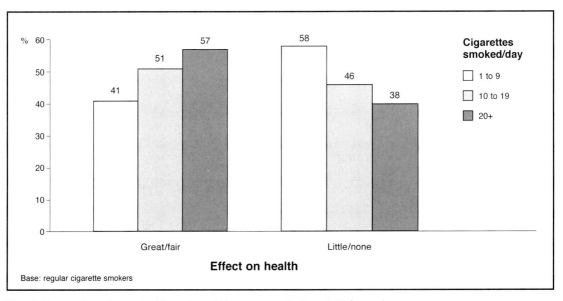

Mantel–Haenszel test for trend with number of cigarettes smoked p < 0.05 for each

(ii) Women

Fig. 3.29. Percentage distribution of smokers' perception of how smoking affects their health by number of cigarettes smoked per day by gender

Table 3.10. Percentage distribution of smokers' perceptions of the way in which smoking affects their health by gender[1]

	Men (%)	Women (%)[2]
Breathlessness	42	41
Coughing	24	24
Wheezing	6	8
Get asthma/make asthma worse	4	6
Prone to chest infections	14	16
Less fit than I used to be	19	12†
Worry about serious illness	6	5
Likely to suffer from cancer	12	8†
Likely to suffer from another serious illness	14	8†
General poor health	7	9
Other[3]	17	17
Don't know/no answer	5	9†
Base:[4]	614	552

[1]Q217 In what ways would you say your smoking affects your health?
[2]Chi-squared test for differences between men and women statistically significant p < 0.05 if marked †
[3]Other includes tiredness, cardiovascular problems, lung disease, sore throats, colds and worse
[4]Base: regular cigarette smokers who answered that smoking affects their health a great deal/fair amount or just a little

The Health and Lifestyle Survey 1992 asked whether respondents thought it was likely that they personally could contract heart disease or lung cancer in the future. About 20% thought they were likely to get heart disease and about 30% thought they were likely to get lung cancer in the future. Blaxter (1990) found that 'cough' was one of the symptoms making up the illness score which smokers commonly declared. West (1995) found that smokers saw the main benefits of giving up as an improvement to current health status and saving money. Prevention of serious illness in the future did not appear to be a strong influence on people.

Smokers' perception of the effect smoking has on their health was broken down by the number of cigarettes smoked a day (Figure 3.30(i)/(ii)). At any level of consumption, breathlessness, followed by coughing was the major effect on health perceived by respondents. Only for women was there any difference in perception of health effects, and only for breathlessness. Heavy smokers were not any more likely to be concerned about the long-term effects of smoking than those who smoked fewer cigarettes. Further analysis of data by age range and occupational group showed little differences between levels of cigarette consumption on perception of effects on health.

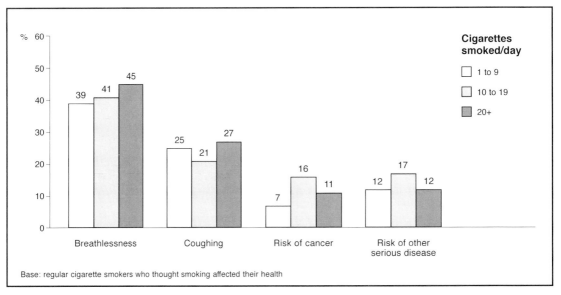

Mantel–Haenszel test for trend with number of cigarettes smoked not statistically significant

(i) Men

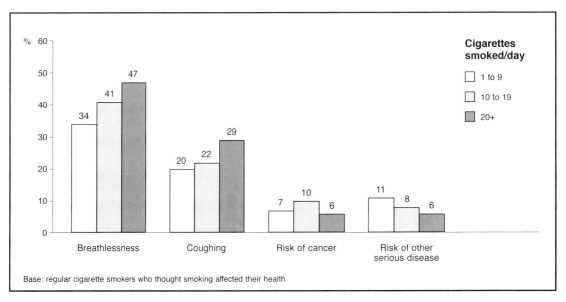

Mantel–Haenszel test for trend with number of cigarettes $p < 0.05$ for breathlessness only

(ii) Women

Fig. 3.30. Percentage distribution of smokers' perception of the effect smoking has on their health by number of cigarettes smoked a day by gender

Perceived effects of passive smoking

All respondents were asked how much, if at all, they would say that passive smoking affected people who were exposed to it (Table 3.11). The majority of men and women reported that passive smoking affected people who were exposed to it a great deal or a fair amount. All the differences between men and women, for each perceived effect, were statistically significant.

Table 3.11. Percentage distribution of the perceived effect of passive smoking by gender[1]

	Men (%)	Women (%)[2]
A great deal	33	41
A fair amount	33	36
Just a little	14	10
Not at all	5	3
It depends	4	2
Don't know/no answer	11	8
Base:	2 754	2 799

[1]Q218 How much, if at all, would you say passive smoking affects people who are exposed to it?
[2]Chi-squared test for differences between men and women statistically significant p < 0.05 for all

Those respondents who thought passive smoking affected health at all were asked in what way would they say passive smoking affected people's health using the same response categories as for active smoking.

Respondents' perceived effects of passive smoking were analysed by the respondents' smoking status (Figure 3.31(i)/(ii)). More cigarette smokers reported 'little/no effect' or 'it depends/don't know' than non-smokers about how much passive smoking affected people's health. Never smokers were nearly twice as likely as current smokers to believe that passive smoking affected other people a great deal (80% compared with 42%). All the differences between smoking status groups were statistically significant except for never versus ex-smokers for great/fair in women and it depends/I don't know for men and women.

When the perceived effects of passive smoking were analysed by age group (Figure 3.32(i)/(ii)) more older people reported that it depends/don't know about the effects of passive smoking than younger people (19% compared with 8%). Younger people were more likely than older people to perceive that passive smoking affected other people (men – younger 76%; older 62%; women – younger 81%; older 74%). Further analysis of the data by occupational group showed only small differences in the responses between groups.

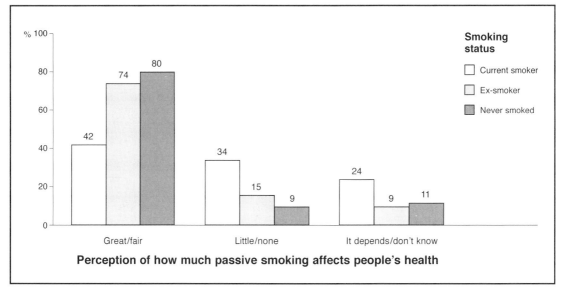

Chi-squared test for differences between smoking categories all p < 0.05 except:
Never versus ex-smokers – it depends/don't know

(i) Men

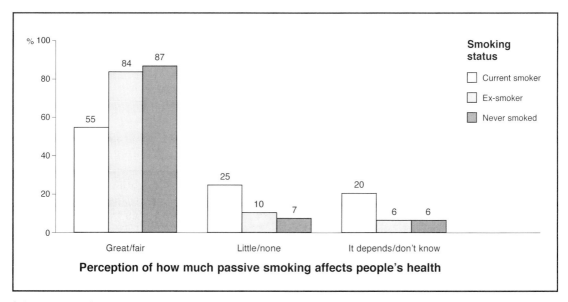

Chi-squared test for differences between smoking categories all p < 0.05 except:
Never versus ex-smokers for great/fair and it depends/don't know

(ii) Women

Fig. 3.31. Percentage distribution of respondents' perception of how passive smoking affects people's health by respondents' smoking status by gender

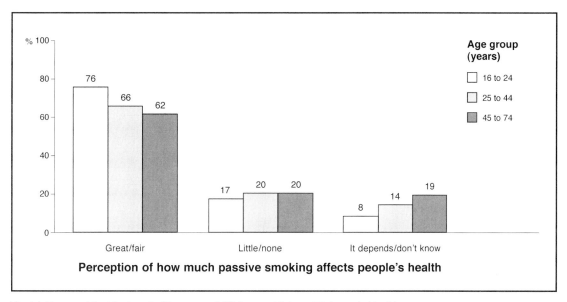

Mantel–Haenszel test for trend with age p < 0.05 for great/fair and it depends/don't know

(i) Men

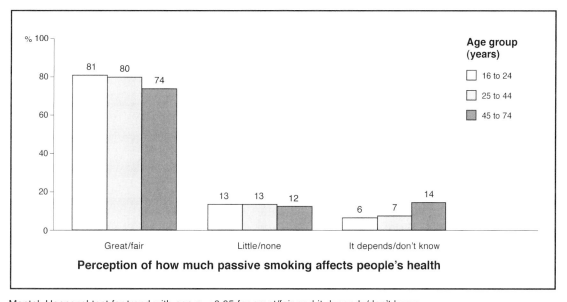

Mantel–Haenszel test for trend with age p < 0.05 for great/fair and it depends/don't know

(ii) Women

Fig. 3.32. Percentage distribution of respondents' perception of the effect of passive smoking on health by age group by gender

Where there was a smoker in the household parents were asked how much, if at all, they thought the health of their child/children was affected by people smoking in the home (Table 3.12). Thirty-nine per cent of men and 37% of women thought that the health of their children was not affected at all. Few thought that smoking affected their children a great deal (5% for men, 9% for women).

Table 3.12. Percentage distribution of the perceived effect on the health of respondents' children by people smoking in the home by gender[1]

	Men (%)	Women (%)[2]
A great deal	5	9
A fair amount	14	20
Just a little	32	23
Not at all	39	37 *
Don't know/no answer	10	10 *
Base:[3]	342	449

[1]Q223 How much, if at all, do you think the health of your child/children is affected by people smoking in the home?
[2]Chi-squared test for differences between men and women statistically significant p < 0.05 unless marked *
[3]Base: parents of children under 16 years with a smoker in the household

Parents who had children under the age of 16 years of age were asked whether they thought parental smoking makes children more likely or less likely to smoke, or has no effect on children starting to smoke (Table 3.13). Fifty-seven per cent of men and 43% of women felt that parental smoking made children more likely to smoke. Those parents with smokers in the household who think smoking in the home affected their children's health were asked: In what ways do you think people smoking in the home affects the health of your child/children? Twenty-six per cent of respondents said breathlessness, 21% prone to chest infections and 23% did not know or did not answer. Parents who smoked were asked whether they thought the fact that they smoked made their child/children more or less likely to smoke or made no difference (Table 3.14). Thirty-one per cent of men and 22% of women perceived that their smoking would mean it was more likely for their children to smoke and 16% of men and 26% of women thought their children would be less likely to smoke. These differences between men and women were statistically significant.

Children whose parents both smoked are two-and-a-half times more likely to smoke than children of non-smoking parents (Department of Health, 1994b). While there may also be demographic, cultural, situational and genetic influences operating on both parents and children, it does identify that children of smoking parents are at higher risk of starting smoking. However the majority of parents do not appear to recognise this increased risk.

Table 3.13. Percentage distribution of parents' perceived effect of parental smoking on the likelihood of children starting to smoke by gender[1]

	Men (%)	Women (%)[2]
More likely	57	43
Less likely	5	11
No difference	28	32 *
It depends	4	5 *
Don't know/no answer	6	9
Base:[3]	826	944

[1]Q225 Do you think parental smoking makes children more likely, less likely to smoke or does it make no difference?
[2]Chi-squared test for differences between men and women statistically significant p < 0.05 unless marked *
[3]Base: parents of children under 16

Table 3.14. Percentage distribution among parents who smoke of the perceived effect of their smoking on the likelihood of their children starting to smoke by gender[1]

	Men (%)	Women (%)[2]
More likely	31	22 †
Less likely	16	26 †
No difference	44	41
It depends	3	6
Don't know/no answer	6	5
Base:[3]	263	289

[1]Q226 Do you think the fact that you smoke makes your child/children more likely, less likely to smoke or does it make no difference?
[2]Chi-squared test for differences between men and women statistically significant p < 0.05 if marked†
[3]Base: parents of children under 16 years who smoke

Discussion

Smoking rates are particularly high for single mothers, those in younger, low-income families and in rented accommodation. Separated or divorced women also have higher rates of smoking, and smokers are more likely to live with other smokers. The King's Fund report on tackling inequalities in health (Benzeval, Judge and Whitehead, 1995) stated that health education and cessation advice has had a limited impact on disadvantaged social groups, which appears to be borne out by this survey. They postulate that health promotion would be more effective if it was more sensitive to the pressures of life for these individuals and backed up with wider social policies and supportive environments. They call for new resources to be invested in developing and evaluating innovative interventions in health education advice and cessation support, particularly by primary care workers, to be targeted at vulnerable groups. Given the high rates in these groups it is clear that there needs to be a continued and more focused strategy of encouraging smokers to attempt to quit, and to provide support through the process. More women in manual occupations fail in their attempts to stop; and women living with a smoker, and smokers in younger, low-income families are less likely to try to stop, and to be successful if they do attempt it. Primary care still provides opportunities to support disadvantaged smokers, but the approaches used need to be more sensitive to the processes of behaviour change and the barriers to change that smokers face. Client-centred approaches to supporting behavioural change in smoking and other risk behaviours, such as those based on the stage of change theory (Prochaska and DiClemente, 1986) may be more effective. While traditional advice-giving methods may be helpful for those people who are ready to take action or are maintaining change, they appear to be less effective for those who have not yet decided to change. These people are either unaware of the risk, or insufficiently motivated by their knowledge to act upon it, in Prochaska and DiClemente's terminology they are either precontemplative or contemplative. For these individuals behavioural counselling that aims, not to change behaviour directly, but to tip the balance of the scales for the individual in favour of thinking about wanting to change may be more effective. This approach requires primary care staff, particularly practice nurses, to learn new client-centred skills, and not to expect success, measured by compliance with health advice, immediately. It is possible that lack of change in the target groups most likely to need it is related to the limitations of current advice-giving processes, and that the more sensitive client-centred approach currently being advocated in courses such as Helping People Change may yield better results, albeit possibly over a longer timescale. This view was endorsed in the King's Fund Centre's seminar on the way forward in cardiovascular disease prevention in primary care (Sharp, 1995).

Given the finding that women living with a smoker are less successful at giving up smoking, primary care workers should consider ways of encouraging partners to try to give up together. This is by no means an easy task, as the Family Heart Study (1994) found; and there are no simple answers to how a women can encourage a reluctant partner to agree to stop smoking. At the least primary care workers should be aware of the particular difficulties women face in this regard, and help them develop strategies to resist these additional counter pressures in their cessation attempts.

In order to provide more support to those on low incomes wishing to stop smoking, Benzeval, Judge and Whitehead (1995) suggest that nicotine replacement therapy (NRT) should be free on prescription for people living on benefits. The authors note that there is some indication that attempts at withdrawal, or simply the knowledge of the health risks of smoking are themselves stress inducing. One of the commonest reasons cited by health care workers for not emphasising smoking cessation with disadvantaged groups is their dependence on cigarettes to cope with stress. The Audit Commission report on coronary heart disease notes that health staff in poorly performing districts argue that socially disadvantaged people need to smoke (Audit Commission, 1995). Although the current cost of over-the-counter sales of nicotine replacement therapies may well prohibit their use by those on low incomes, there may also be an important role for pharmacy staff to play in smoking cessation. Training for pharmacists and their staff in smoking cessation may contribute to the successful use of NRT. The survey showed that manual workers, and those in the cluster group of younger, low-income families were more likely to start smoking before the age of 16. Also, the older both men and women are when they start smoking, the more likely they are to be able to give up later on, most often between the ages of 25 and 34. The fewer cigarettes people smoke, again the more likely they are to be able to give up. It would seem then that the most success would be with men and women in their twenties or early thirties, who are not heavy smokers. Health care workers may feel that this group is less at risk, has fewer smoking-related health problems; or because they are more able to give up, should not be given as much support as older, heavier smokers. In fact they may well be more responsive to prompts to act and more ready to follow cessation advice.

There is evidence that school-based health education programmes can delay the onset of smoking (Dent *et al.*, 1995). As very few people over the age of 20 start to smoke, there would appear to be benefit from focusing smoking prevention with young people on the advantages of delaying starting smoking, rather than on not smoking at all. Providing the information about relative ease of cessation with later starting and lighter habit may provide an easier choice for some young people than not smoking altogether. It may be easier to think that one will try it one day, but not now, rather than never smoke at all. This type of 'harm minimisation' approach is advocated for some aspects of substance misuse, and recognises the reality of the context in which young people live and in which health education messages may seem entirely irrelevant. This type of message may be more meaningful to young people in secondary education. It is also the responsibility of the tertiary education sector to maintain health education interventions about smoking prevention. As most secondary-school students transfer to sixth-form colleges, and as increasingly large numbers of students are progressing to higher education, there are real opportunities to continue the attempt to delay students starting to smoke in these settings.

Enforcement of the Children and Young Persons (Protection from Tobacco) Act 1991, which makes it illegal to sell any tobacco product to anyone below the age of 16, would also contribute to preventing children starting to smoke. A 1994 OPCS survey found that only 13% of children were unable to buy cigarettes the last time they tried (Diamond, 1995). Prosecutions and convictions have, however, risen since the introduction of the Act, and the law appears to be enforced more rigorously in areas where child volunteers are used to make test purchases of cigarettes (Foulds and Godfrey, 1995). Guidelines are available for trading standards officers explaining how the law can be enforced (HEA, 1994). Townsend (1995) calls for an increase in the legal age for buying cigarettes to 18, in line with the minimum age for buying alcohol, as a further contribution to delaying uptake of smoking.

Much of the above has focused on attempts to improve health promotion with individuals; however it is increasingly recognised that providing supportive environments has a considerable part to play both in encouraging cessation attempts, and in reducing the numbers of cigarettes consumed. In smoking prevention most attention has been paid to introducing smoking policies banning, or limiting, smoking in public places. Whilst recent surveys by the CBI and Reed Personnel Services have indicated 85–86% of employers have a smoking policy, this is more apparent with larger companies. However it is unclear how many small companies, and those employing mainly manual workers have smoking limitations. Smoking restrictions in restaurants have become more commonplace, and this survey shows that the majority of smokers feel they should not smoke in restaurants, but fewer younger people agreed. Of concern is the finding that smokers in younger, low-income families and the older less-educated smokers are more likely to ignore smoking bans. In countries such as the USA and France where total bans in public places have been variously imposed, there are widespread signs of flouting the rules and growing opposition, particularly from restaurateurs who may be losing business. Despite the more general acceptance of smoking bans in society as a whole, there is a need to ensure that these are continuing to be introduced with sensitivity and with the acceptance of users of services, particularly where these are the more disadvantaged in society. All sections of the population clearly accept the need to avoid smoking near babies, children and pregnant women. Conversely this study showed that most people, whether or not they were smokers, were tolerant and permissive of visitors smoking in their homes. It would appear that it would not be acceptable at the moment to attempt to influence the social norms about smoking in private homes. For most this would probably be seen as an invasion of privacy and an imposition of unsociable behaviour.

Older people, and men and women in manual occupations appear to be less aware of, or able to accept, the need for women to stop smoking in pregnancy. This indicates a continued need for those working with pregnant women and their families to point out the health risks and offer cessation advice. There might also be value in educational campaigns directed at older people as grandparents emphasising their support to helping their daughters give up when pregnant. Parents who smoke do not seem to be aware of, or are not prepared to admit, the effects of their smoking on the health of their children. Whilst about a half of all parents were aware that parental smoking made children more likely to smoke, this figure dropped substantially to only a third of fathers and a fifth of mothers who smoked. Of concern is the finding that one in six fathers who smoked, and one in four mothers, thought that their smoking would make their children *less* likely to smoke. It would appear that there is still a need to inform parents about the evidence linking parents' smoking with an increased likelihood of their children starting to smoke.

Finally the effect of the above initiatives would probably be enhanced by banning the advertising of tobacco products.* This has been widely debated but its disproportional effect on socially disadvantaged smokers has not been adequately stressed. As advertising is more predominant in poorer areas, in the tabloid press and in young people's magazines, Townsend (1995) notes that an advertising ban might well have most effect on people with low incomes and on recruitment to smoking at young ages.

*At the time of writing, legislation may be necessary for a limited ban on tobacco sponsorship of sport and advertising.

References

Audit Commission (1995). *Dear to our hearts? Commissioning service for treatment and prevention of coronary heart disease.* London: HMSO.

Bennett, N, Dodd, T, Flatley, J, Freeth, S and Bolling, K (1995). *Health survey for England 1993.* London: HMSO.

Benzeval, M, Judge, K and Whitehead, M (1995). *Tackling inequalities in health: an agenda for action.* London: King's Fund.

Blackburn, C and Graham, H (1992). *Smoking among working class mothers.* Department of Applied Social Studies, University of Warwick.

Blaxter, M (1990). *Health and lifestyle.* London: Tavistock/Routledge.

Buck, D and Godfrey, C (1994). *Helping smokers give up: guidance for purchasers on cost-effectiveness.* London: Health Education Authority.

Cardozo, L, Gobb, D, Studd, J and Copper, D (1982). Social and obstetric factors associated with smoking in pregnancy. *British Journal of Obstetrics and Gynaecology* **99**:22–7.

Cox, B D, Blaxter, M, Buckle, A L J, Fenner, N P, Roth, Sir M, Start, J, Wadsworth, M E J and

Whichelow, M (1987). *Lifestyle survey: preliminary report.* London: Health Promotion Research Trust.

Dent, J W, Sussman, S, Stacy, A W, Craig, S, Burton, D and Flay, D R (1995). Two-year behaviour outcomes of project towards no tobacco use. *Journal of Consulting and Clinical Psychology* **63**:676–7.

Department of Health (1992). *The health of the nation: a strategy for health in England.* London: HMSO.

Department of Health (1994a). *National Opinion Poll – smoking habits.* Unpublished.

Department of Health (1994b). *Smokefree for health: an action plan to achieve the Health of the Nation targets.* London: HMSO.

Diamond, A (1995). *Smoking among secondary schoolchildren in 1994.* London: HMSO.

Family Heart Study Group (1994). Randomised control trial evaluating cardiovascular screening and intervention in general practice: principal results of British family heart study. *British Medical Journal* **308**:313–20.

Foulds, J and Godfrey, C (1995). Counting the costs of children's smoking. *British Medical Journal* **311**:1152–3.

Health Education Authority (1994). *Not for sale – stopping smoking before it starts.* London: HEA.

Health Education Authority and MORI (1995). *A survey of the UK population, Part 1.* London: HEA.

Jarvis, M J and Jackson, P (1988). Cigar and pipe smoking in Britain: implications for smoking prevalence and cessation. *British Journal of Addiction* **83**:323–30.

Marsh, A and McKay, S (1994). *Poor smokers.* London: Policy Studies Institute.

Prochaska, J and DiClemente, C (1986). Toward a comprehensive model of change. In: Miller, W R and Heather, N (eds) *Treating addictive behaviors: processes of change.* New York: Plenum.

Sharp, I (ed.) (1995). *Preventing coronary heart disease in primary care: the way forward.* National Heart Forum. London: HMSO.

Thomas, M, Goddard, E, Hickman, M and Hunter, P (1994). *General household survey 1992.* London: HMSO.

Townsend, J (1995). The burden of smoking. In: Benzeval, M, Judge, K and Whitehead, M *Tackling inequalities in health: an agenda for action.* London: King's Fund.

West, R (1995). *Escaping the nicotine trap.* London: HEA.

4. Nutrition

Introduction

This chapter summarises the main results from the analysis of the nutrition data. It is presented in three sections: knowledge about diet and eating, sources of learning about cooking and levels of information about cholesterol. As with the previous section, as well as presenting the detailed data, the analysis attempts to explore the important interactions in order to identify which groups are eating less healthily and to understand some of the constraints on dietary behaviour.

- Most respondents considered they knew something about how to reduce people's risk of heart disease, but relatively fewer knew about how people could reduce their risk of diabetes, stroke, and particularly osteoporosis. Few people seemed to know about the benefits of exercise on risk of osteoporosis.

- Women were more likely than men to believe people could reduce their risk of disease.

- Respondents defined by cluster analysis to be middle-aged educated were more likely to believe people could reduce their risk of disease than those in the younger, low-income families cluster.

- Although respondents felt reasonably confident explaining about fats in general, most were not confident to explain about types of fat or E numbers; men less so than women. Respondents in the middle-aged, educated cluster were more likely to think that foods high in fat were high in fat compared with subjects in the cluster grouping older less-educated respondents.

- There were some inconsistencies in people's knowledge about the fat content of margarine compared with butter; although the questionnaire did not differentiate between the many varieties of margarine available, many people incorrectly thought margarine was low in fat.

- Even respondents who felt confident about explaining about fats were confused about the fat content of margarine.

- Nearly half of the respondents felt well informed about cholesterol and most had correct knowledge about a series of statements about cholesterol.

- There were considerable demographic group differences in people's knowledge about cholesterol and the saturated fat content of foods; those who felt well informed about saturated fats were more likely to get the answers to questions right; non-manual subjects were better informed than those in manual occupations.

Knowledge and learning

This section assesses people's knowledge about diet and its relationship with health and disease and how confident they are about their understanding of certain dietary terms. The relationship between knowledge and confidence is explored and certain misconceptions exposed. Where people learn to cook, and their preference for sources of further information are discussed. Levels of understanding about cholesterol are also considered.

Knowledge

Table 4.1 presents respondents' knowledge about what people can do to reduce their risk of getting heart disease, diabetes, stroke and osteoporosis. For most risk factors over half of the respondents felt that there was something that people could do to reduce their chances of getting heart disease; over 70% of respondents thought that people could reduce their risk by giving up smoking, reducing fat intake, taking regular exercise and controlling body weight (68% in men). Fewer than half of the respondents felt that people could reduce their risk of heart disease by eating plenty of fresh fruit and vegetables, reducing sugar intake or increasing starch and fibre intake. Very few people indicated they did not know of anything people could do to reduce their risk of heart disease.

In comparison with heart disease many fewer people thought there was anything they could do to reduce the chance of diabetes (except reducing sugar intake, 62% and 67% of men and women respectively) and osteoporosis. For stroke, over half the respondents thought people could reduce their risk by reducing stress and also by giving up or reducing smoking. Over 40% of respondents also thought that controlling body weight and reducing fat intake could protect people against stroke. Perhaps surprisingly, for osteoporosis the risk factor which was mentioned by the largest number of subjects (22% and 37% for men and women respectively) was eating a balanced diet. However 58% of men and 40% of women did not know what they could do to reduce their risk of osteoporosis, and 25% of men and 19% of women did not know what could be done to reduce people's risk of diabetes.

For all four disease groups and for most risk factors asked about, women were more likely than men to indicate that people could do something about them. The biggest differences were for risk factors for osteoporosis (exercise: men 12%, women 26% and a balanced diet: men 22%, women 37%). Most of the gender differences were statistically significant except for stroke.

Further demographic comparisons were made to assess whether age, occupation, marital status and geographic region influenced the responses of subjects for each condition separately.

Table 4.1. Percentage distribution of respondents' knowledge of protection against heart disease, diabetes, stroke and osteoporosis by gender[1]

	Heart disease[2]		Diabetes[2]		Stroke[2]		Osteoporosis[2]	
	M(%)	W(%)	M(%)	W(%)	M(%)	W(%)	M(%)	W(%)
Control bodyweight	68	70 *	14	22	43	42 *	10	19
Reduce sugar intake	43	43 *	62	67	20	20 *	4	5
Reduce fat intake	75	79	8	10	41	44 *	6	8
Increase starch and fibre intake	32	35	7	8 *	16	17 *	10	10 *
Eat a balanced diet	59	64	25	28	36	37 *	22	37
Limit alcohol consumption	63	66	20	22 *	38	40 *	6	10
Give up or cut down on smoking	79	84	9	13	52	58	8	15
Eat plenty of fresh fruit and vegetables	47	49	13	16	23	24 *	20	29
Reduce salt intake	50	59	8	12	29	36	7	8
Take regular exercise	72	75	8	10	46	45 *	12	26
Reduce stress	64	68	7	9 *	51	55	4	6
None of these	<1	<1 *	4	4 *	1	1 *	3	3 *
Don't know	2	1	25	19	15	14 *	58	40
Base:	2 754	2 799	2 754	2 799	2 754	2 799	2 754	2 799

[1]Q93 to Q96 Which, if any, of these can people do to reduce their chances of getting heart disease etc. Multiple response question

[2]Chi-squared test for differences between men and women statistically significant p < 0.05 unless marked *

Heart disease

The percentage of males and females who considered that reducing fat intake could reduce people's risk of heart disease was lowest in the oldest age group (58% for men and 68% for women), but similar across other age groups (77% for men and 81% for women). The trend for age was statistically significant. For the other more commonly mentioned risk factors age differences were smaller. Young men and women (16- to 19-year-olds) were the least likely to mention that increasing fruit and vegetable consumption could reduce risk of heart disease (37% for men and 37% for women; gender difference not statistically significant), compared with 47% for men in other age groups combined and 50% in women in other age groups combined (gender difference statistically significant). Respondents employed in manual occupations (men and women) compared with non-manual occupations were less likely to believe that people could reduce their risk of heart disease by reducing fat intake (70% compared with 83%; difference statistically significant), giving up smoking (particularly men 74% compared with 84%; women 81% compared with 88%; manual compared with non-manual respectively), controlling weight (over 80% in professional and managers and around 50% in unskilled manual) or eat more fruit and vegetables (41% in men and 45% in women in manual occupations compared with 53% in men and 53% in non-manual occupations; occupational group differences statistically significant). Widowed men and women (although numbers were small) were much less likely to consider that people could reduce their risk of heart disease by reducing their fat intake (57% for widowed men and 67% for widowed women compared with 75% and 81% respectively for married men and women (marital status differences statistically significant). There were no major regional differences in the responses of subjects.

A further analysis using the demographic clusters suggested that people with qualifications, who are in employment, own their own property, have a car and are living in a two-adult household with children are more likely to suggest that risk can be reduced by altering risk factors (cluster 3 – middle-aged educated); for example, 85% in this group believed reducing fat could reduce people's risk compared with 67% of people in a cluster defined by no formal qualifications, manual occupation, older and retired subjects (cluster 4 – older, less-educated) (Figure 4.1).

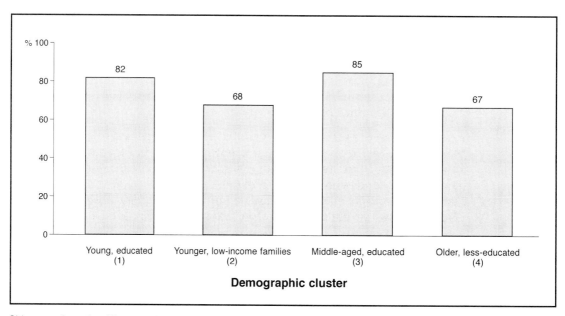

Chi-squared test for differences between clusters p < 0.05 all except 1 v 3, 2 v 4

Fig. 4.1. Percentage of respondents reporting that people can reduce their chances of getting heart disease by reducing fat intake by demographic cluster group

Diabetes

Female respondents in the youngest age group (16–19 years 10%, compared with 23% in other age groups; difference statistically significant) were less likely to consider that controlling body weight was something that people could do to control diabetes. There were no differences for men. For both men and women there were also differences between those employed in manual compared with non-manual occupations in the percentage of respondents believing that people could reduce their risk of diabetes by controlling body weight (men – manual 10%, compared with non-manual 18%; women – manual 19%, compared with non-manual 25%; gender and occupational differences statistically significant). There were no obvious age, marital status, or occupational group differences in the percentage of people who considered reducing sugar intake could decrease people's risk of diabetes.

Stroke

The number of people providing answers limits the reliability of further demographic group specific data. There was a tendency for younger men and women and respondents in non-manual occupations to be less likely than older respondents to consider that reducing salt could lower people's risk of stroke. Other age differences were less obvious for stroke risk factors. There were no other obvious differences between responses broken down by demographic variables.

Osteoporosis

Younger men (15%) and middle-aged women (33%) and non-manual occupational groups (women – non-manual 31%, manual 21%; men – non-manual 14%, manual 10%) were most likely to believe that taking regular exercise could reduce people's risk of osteoporosis.

Using the demographic cluster variable further highlighted differences in beliefs about the benefits of regular exercise; among those people on income support, living in rented accommodation, no car, unemployed, no qualifications and who are single parents (cluster 2 – younger, low-income families) only 13% believed exercise could reduce people's risk, whereas 24% of subjects in the middle-aged, educated cluster believed exercise could reduce risk (Figure 4.2).

People were asked which of a list of topics they would not feel confident explaining to someone else (Table 4.2). For most items over two-thirds of subjects felt that they could explain the topics listed, the exceptions being for types of fat and E numbers. Overall men were less confident than women about explaining all the terms listed, with the largest difference being for types of fat. Nearly half of all men did not feel confident explaining about polyunsaturated fat.

Table 4.2. Percentage distribution of respondents' confidence in explaining terms relating to diet and eating by gender[1]

| | Respondent did not feel confident explaining named term[2] | |
	Men (%)	Women (%)
Cholesterol	28	25
Fibre	14	7
Energy	11	8
Starchy foods	18	9
Fats	12	7
Polyunsaturated fat	48	38
Saturated fat	36	30
A balanced diet	12	7
Carbohydrates	23	15
Calories	13	8
Vitamins	13	8
E number or additives	38	36
Felt confident in explaining all terms	29	33
Don't know/no answer	2	2 *
Base:	2 754	2 799

[1]Q92 These are some terms relating to diet and eating. Which if any of these terms would you not feel confident explaining to someone else? Multiple response question
[2]Chi-squared test for differences between men and women statistically significant $p < 0.05$ unless marked *

Respondents in the younger age groups combined (16 to 24 years) were least likely to feel confident about explaining all of the terms listed (20% men, 20% women, compared with 36% men and 37% women in the 65 to 74 years age group; age differences statistically significant by gender). There was also a divide based on occupational group: respondents employed in non-manual occupations were more likely to feel confident about explaining all terms than respondents in manual occupational groups (36% for women and 33% for non-manual men, compared with 28% and 25% respectively for female and male manual workers; occupational group differences statistically significant).

Subjects were then asked which foods they thought were high in fat and particularly saturated fat (Table 4.3). Responses to this question highlighted some inconsistencies in respondents' knowledge; whereas over 80% of subjects thought butter was high in fat, only 35% of men and 48% of women thought soft margarine was high in fat. Data from the National Food Survey (1994) show that about 23% of fat consumed in 1993 was low fat and dairy spreads. In the present study it is not possible to differentiate between people's knowledge about soft margarine and low-fat spreads; it is likely that for at least a proportion of subjects the fat they use is lower in fat than butter, but there must still be an important group of people who are misinformed about the fat content of margarine products, and in relation to butter.

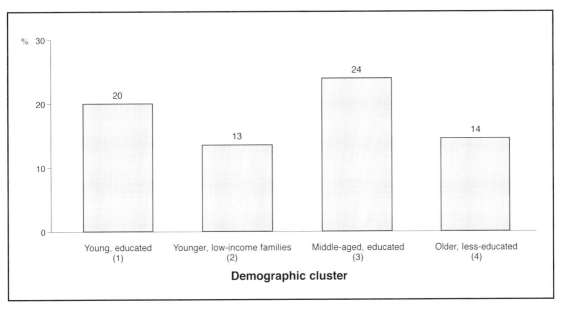

Chi-squared test for differences between clusters p < 0.05 except for 2 v 4

Fig. 4.2. Percentage of respondents reporting that people can reduce their chances of getting osteoporosis by taking regular exercise by demographic cluster group

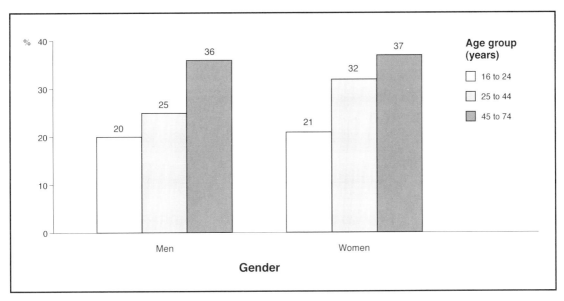

Mantel–Haenszel test for trend with age p < 0.05 for men and women

Fig. 4.3. Percentage of respondents feeling confident to explain all the terms in Table 4.2 by age group by gender

Table 4.3. Percentage distribution of respondents' knowledge about fat and saturated fat content of foods by gender[1]

	Fat[2]		Saturated fat[2]	
	Men (%)	Women (%)	Men (%)	Women (%)
Red meat	47	47 *	27	29 *
Chicken	6	4	3	2
White fish (not fried)	1	1 *	2	1 *
Pies, pasties, quiches	47	58	30	35
Pasta and noodles	8	5	4	4 *
Potatoes (not chips)	4	4 *	2	3 *
Whole milk	63	68	32	36
Cheese	73	79	41	44
Soft margarine	35	48	24	34
Fruit	1	2	1	1 *
Butter	81	84	51	56
Crisps	54	65	32	37
Biscuits	38	50	20	26
None of these	<1	<1 *	1	<1 *
Don't know/no answer	4	2	27	21
Base:	2 754	2 799	2 754	2 799

[1]Q97 Which of the following foods on this card do you think are high in fat or saturated fat? Multiple response question
[2]Chi-squared test for differences between men and women statistically significant $p < 0.05$ unless marked *

Nearly two-thirds of respondents thought milk was high in fat; while full-fat milk is a major contributor to total fat intake, it has about 4 grams of fat per 100 grams, compared with 21 grams of fat per 100 grams in a steak and kidney pie. Low-fat milk accounts for more than half of milk and cream consumption in the UK, with an occupational gradient to higher low-fat milk consumption in non-manual occupational groups (National Food Survey, 1994). Few people considered chicken to be high in fat; the fat content of chicken varies depending on preparation and serving methods and the fat content can vary from 4 grams per 100 grams to over 20 grams per 100 grams (Holland et al., 1991). Nearly half of all respondents felt that red meat, pies and pasties, crisps and biscuits (38% in men, 50% in women) were high in fat. Few people considered pasta and potatoes had a high fat content.

Respondents' knowledge about the fat content of foods was compared for the demographic clusters (Figure 4.5). For all the foods presented in Figure 4.5 respondents in younger, low-income families and older and less-educated (clusters 2 and 4) were less likely to think they were high in fat compared particularly with middle-aged educated respondents and young, educated respondents (clusters 3 and 1). About a third of older, less-educated respondents thought that red meat, soft margarine, and biscuits were high in fat compared with about 50% of middle-aged educated respondents.

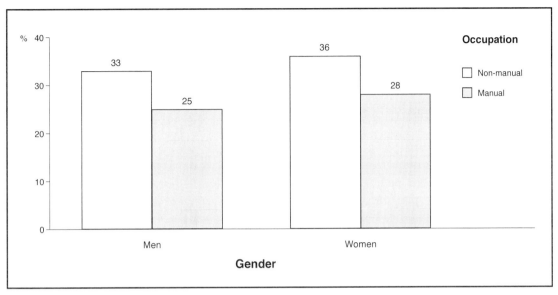

Chi-squared test for differences between occupational groups p < 0.05 for men and women

Fig. 4.4. Percentage of respondents feeling confident to explain all the terms in Table 4.2 by occupational group by gender

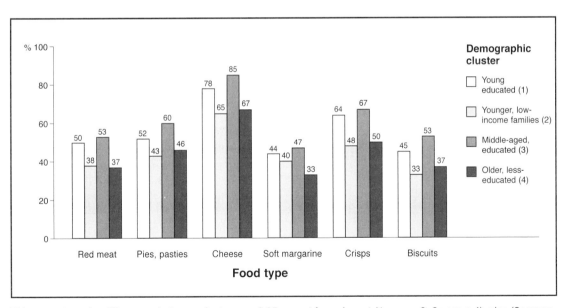

Chi-squared test for differences between clusters p < 0.05 except for red meat (1 versus 3, 2 versus 4), pies (2 versus 4), cheese (2 versus 4), soft margarine (1 versus 2), crisps (2 versus 4), biscuits (2 versus 4)

Fig. 4.5. Percentage of respondents thinking each food group is high in fat by demographic cluster group

Many fewer subjects thought that red meat, pies, whole milk, cheese, margarine, butter and crisps were high in saturated fats as compared with total fat. It is not possible from the answers to these questions to determine whether respondents were describing the composition of foods or the contribution that food makes to the overall diet; certain foods may have a high fat content but are rarely eaten and so are not a major source of fat in a usual diet.

The relationship between how confident people felt about explaining terms and their knowledge about the fat content of selected foods was explored further (Figure 4.6(i)/(ii)). Overall about 88% of men and 93% of women felt confident explaining about fats to someone else (Table 4.2). Thirty-five per cent of men and 48% of women thought that margarine was high in fat, as against 81% and 84% for butter (it would be expected that the percentages for butter and margarine would be similar). Among those who were confident in explaining about fats, only 36% of men and 49% of women correctly believed margarine was high in fat. Among those few people who were not confident only 28% of men and 37% of women believed margarine was high in fat. Younger (under 45 years of age) men and women (men – younger 39%, older 31%; women – younger 54%, older 44%) and those employed in non-manual occupations were more likely to correctly believe margarine was high in fat (men – non-manual 38%, manual 33%; women – non-manual 53%, manual 45%). All of the above comparisons were statistically significant. This indicates that particularly older men and women in manual occupations have inaccurate knowledge about fats.

The relationship between confidence and knowledge for fat content of pies,

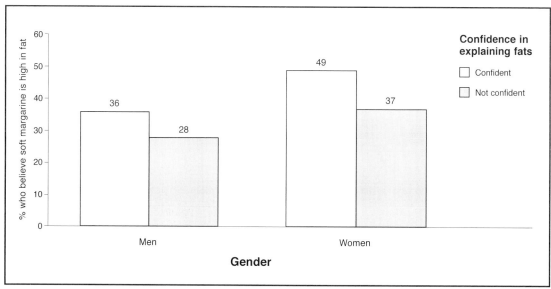

Chi-squared test for differences between those who are confident and those not confident $p < 0.05$ for men and women

(i) Soft margarine

Fig. 4.6. Percentage distribution of respondents' confidence in explaining fats and belief that selected foods are high in fat by gender

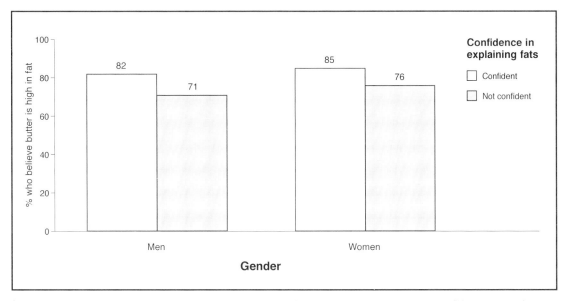

Chi-squared test for differences between those who were confident and those who were not confident p < 0.05 for men and women

(ii) Butter

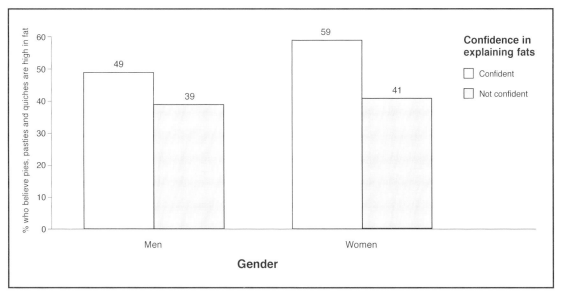

Chi-squared test for differences between those who were confident and those who were not confident p < 0.05 for men and women

(iii) Pies, pasties and quiches

Fig. 4.6. Percentage distribution of respondents' confidence in explaining fats and belief that selected foods are high in fat by gender

pasties and quiches is explored in Figure 4.6(iii). Respondents who felt they were more confident were more likely to accurately believe that these foods were high in fats than those respondents who were not confident. Women in this group were more likely to be correct than men. The differences in the percentage of confident subjects and those who were not confident were also apparent when assessed by age and occupational groups. Younger men and women, and those employed in manual occupations who were not confident about explaining about fats, were the least likely to say that pies etc. were high in fats.

Sources of learning about cooking

Respondents were asked where they first learnt about cooking and where they learnt from later on (Table 4.4). Most men and women began to learn about cooking from their mother, more so for women than men. For women, schools and cookery books were also important sources of learning about cooking. Younger respondents, particularly males, were more likely to have initially learnt about cooking from their mothers than older respondents (for men 69% aged 16–24 years compared with 48% for men aged 45–74 years) (Figure 4.7). Men in manual occupations compared with those in non-manual occupations (10% compared with 20%) were less likely to have learnt initially using cookery books.

Later in life more respondents considered cookery books to be a source of learning, followed by cookery programmes on television and, particularly for women, articles in magazines/newspapers. The older the respondent the less likely their mother was considered to be a source of later learning. (Men – 16–24 years 27%, 25–44 years 10%; women – 16–24 years 28%, 25–44 years 12%, age trends statistically significant.) Men and women in non-manual occupations were more likely to prefer books as a source of later learning, than manual workers (men – non-manual 37%, manual 23%; women – non-manual 59%, manual 53%). Older women were also more likely to prefer books (16–24 years 45%; 25–44 years 59%). All of the comparisons between age, and occupational groups for each gender were statistically significant.

About half of all respondents (49% of men and 52% of women) answered yes when asked if they would like to learn more about cooking. When asked what sources of information they would use to find out more about cooking 57% of men and 54% of women would prefer to use cookery books; 34% of men and 38% of women would prefer cookery programmes on television; 23% of men and 36% of women mentioned cookery classes, and 33% of men and 22% of women said they would prefer asking a member of their family. Sixteen per cent or less of subjects said they would prefer leaflets from supermarkets or articles in magazines. Older men and women (men – 16–24 years 26%, 45–74 years 36%; women – 16–24 years 28%, 45–74 years 44%, age trend statistically significant by gender) were more likely to prefer television as a source of learning. Men and women living with a partner were also more likely to prefer television than those living without a partner (men – with partner 40%, without partner 25%; women – with partner 42%, without partner 31%); differences were statistically significant.

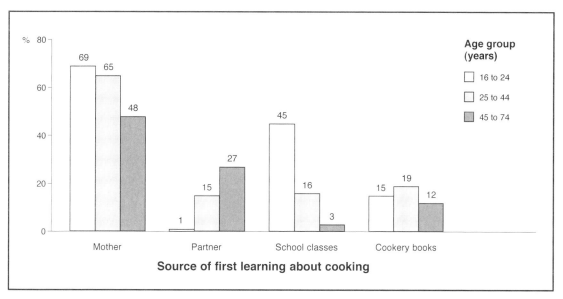

Mantel–Haenszel test for trend with age p < 0.05 for all sources

(i) Men

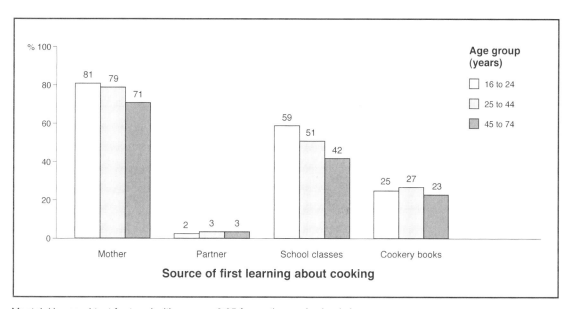

Mantel–Haenszel test for trend with age p < 0.05 for mother and school classes

(ii) Women

Fig. 4.7. Percentage distribution of source of learning when first started learning to cook by age group by gender

Table 4.4. Percentage distribution of respondents' sources of learning about cooking when first started to cook and later on by gender[1]

	First learnt[2]		Later learnt[2]	
	Men (%)	Women (%)	Men (%)	Women (%)
Mother	58	76	11	13
Father	11	6	2	2 [‡]
Grandmother	7	13	2	2 *
Wife/husband/partner	18	3	26	5
Other relatives	5	7	5	6 *
Friends	9	7	10	11 *
Childminder	<1	<1 †	0	<1
Cookery classes at school	15	49	4	15
Other cookery courses	2	4	3	8
Cookery books	15	25	30	56
Cookery programmes on TV	5	4 *	15	24
Specialist cookery/food magazines	1	3	4	9
Articles in magazines/ newspapers	2	5	8	23
Leaflets from supermarkets	1	2 *	6	11
Leaflets from food producers	1	1 *	3	5
Health centre/doctor	<1	<1 *	1	1 *
None of these	5	1	15	7
Don't know	1	<1	3	2
Haven't learnt to cook	8	1	8	1
Base: all	2 754	2 799	2 754	2 799

[1] Sources of learning Q134 when first started cooking, Q135 later. Multiple response questions
[2] Chi-squared test for differences between men and women statistically significant $p < 0.05$ unless marked *
† Actual figures 0.1% and 0.4% for men and women respectively
‡ Actual figures 2.3% and 1.5% for men and women respectively

Information levels about cholesterol

Respondents were asked how well informed they felt about cholesterol (Table 4.5). Forty-eight per cent of men and 50% of women felt either fairly or very well informed about cholesterol. Older male and female respondents and those in non-manual occupational groups were more likely to feel better informed than younger people and those employed in manual occupations (age data; non-manual, manual data; all comparisons statistically significant). Subjects from younger, low-income families (cluster group 2) were very much more likely to feel not at all informed than middle-aged educated respondents (cluster group 3), (20% in cluster 2 compared with 6% in cluster 3).

Table 4.5. Percentage distribution of how well informed respondents felt about cholesterol by gender[1]

	Men (%)	Women (%)[2]
Very well informed	11	10
Fairly well informed	37	40 †
Not very well informed	37	39
Not at all informed	13	10 †
Don't know/no answer	2	2
Base:	2 754	2 799

[1]Q147 How well informed do you feel about cholesterol?
[2]Chi-squared test for differences between men and women statistically significant p < 0.05 marked †

Subjects were then given a series of statements and asked which were true (Table 4.6). The overwhelming majority got the right answers, except for the statement about one type of cholesterol in the blood being called serum cholesterol. It is not clear why this question was so badly answered because it appeared from other answers that they understood about treatment for high blood cholesterol. About 30% of subjects wrongly believed that cholesterol only comes from the foods that are eaten. Thirty-one per cent of men and 25% of women answered wrongly to the question about blood cholesterol being lowered by eating a diet low in saturated fat.

Overall about 15% of respondents answered don't know to the above question about cholesterol. When broken down by the demographic cluster variable, 27% of subjects in younger, low-income families (cluster 2) answered that they don't know compared with only 7% in the middle-aged educated group (cluster 3). For the question about high blood cholesterol being able to be reduced by a diet low in saturated fat, older, less-educated respondents (cluster 4) were much more likely to think this was not true than middle-aged educated respondents (cluster 3), (cluster 4, 62%; cluster 3, 82%).

The relationship between perceived and actual knowledge about cholesterol was explored further; 81% of men and 84% of women who felt well informed answered the question correctly about the effects of a diet low in saturated fat (question 1 in Table 4.6), compared with 59% in men and 67% in women who did not feel well informed (differences statistically significant). Respondents in non-manual occupations, whether they thought they were well informed or not, were more likely to get the right answer to this question than respondents in manual occupations (men – non-manual 82%, manual 59%; women – non-manual 80%, manual 67%; gender specific differences statistically significant). Age did not appear to influence the relationship between perceived and actual knowledge.

Table 4.6. Percentage distribution of respondents' knowledge about cholesterol by gender[1]

	% respondents who answered correctly[2]	
	Men	Women
1. High blood cholesterol can be reduced by eating a diet low in saturated fat[3]	69	75
2. People only get raised cholesterol levels if it runs in their family	93	91
3. Low cholesterol causes cancer	99	99 *
4. Cholesterol only comes from the foods you eat	68	71
5. One type of cholesterol in the blood is called serum cholesterol[3]	10	10 *
6. Only people with high blood pressure have high cholesterol	94	94 *
7. High blood cholesterol can only be reduced by taking medication (drugs)	91	89
8. None of these	2	2 *
9. Don't know/no answer	16	14
Base:	2 754	2 799

[1]Q150 Which if any of these statements describe cholesterol? Tell me all those you think are true
[2]Chi-squared test for differences between men and women statistically significant $p < 0.05$ unless marked *
[3]Statements are correct; all others are incorrect

Dietary and eating patterns

This section reviews the dietary patterns of the respondents and identifies those eating more or less healthy diets by cluster analysis. Eating and shopping practices are also explored.

- Many people in all socio-demographic clusters are eating 'less healthy' diets, but two-thirds of the younger, low-income families were eating less healthy diets.

- Cost is a major factor in influencing where people shop and what they buy.

- Socio-demographic differences highlight the need for a more targeted approach for messages aimed at improving dietary practices, which takes account of people's income and access to shops.

- The men who are most likely to benefit from dietary change (manual workers) are the groups least likely to eat lunch in a workplace canteen. One-half of male manual workers eat a packed lunch from home. The reverse is true for women, with more in non-manual occupations eating a packed lunch.

Dietary patterns

The DINE questionnaire developed in Oxford was used in this study to assess dietary intakes. Subjects were asked how often they ate foods grouped into the following categories: bread, breakfast cereals, starchy foods and fruit and vegetables, meat, cheese, fried foods, cakes and biscuits (Table 4.7). Data from the frequency questionnaire were used to derive a weighted score for fibre, fat and unsaturated fat. On the basis of these scores subjects were grouped into low, moderate or high intakes for fibre, fat and unsaturated fat. This method does not allow gram weights of foods to be estimated, but the method has been shown in a calibration study to correlate well with an absolute measure of intake (Roe *et al.*, 1994). We have also derived an index of fruit consumption.

Most people ate bread every day (1% of men and 2% of women said that they never ate bread). Among those that ate bread, white bread was more commonly eaten than other types (56% of men and 45% of women ate white bread, and 24% of men and 29% of women ate wholemeal bread). These latter figures are comparable to those reported from the Health Survey for England 1993 (Bennett *et al.*, 1995) (25% men and 31% women eating wholemeal bread). Of those eating bread, men were more likely to eat more bread than women (more than 3 slices a day; men 43%; women 15%) (Table 4.7(i)).

Of the 75% of respondents eating breakfast cereal (about 70% in the Health Survey for England 1993), 28% of men and 23% of women ate rice/corn cereals, followed by 20% and 19% for men and women respectively for wheat cereals (Table 4.7(ii)). Few reported eating sugary type cereals.

Over 40% of respondents stated that they ate fruit and vegetables more than six times a week, although among men 13% stated that they ate fruit less than once a week. Most people ate potatoes at least three times a week; with fewer people eating beans and rice and related products more than once a week (Table 4.7(iii)). Most people ate each of the meat items listed less than or equal to once a week (Table 4.7(iv)). Just over 10 per cent of respondents ate cakes/pies/puddings six or more times a week; nearly one-third ate biscuits/chocolates six or more times a week (Table 4.7(v)). About two-thirds of respondents currently consume either skimmed or semi-skimmed milk. Of those consuming milk, most have about a half a pint or more a day (Table 4.7(vi)). More women than men (29% compared with 21%) reported using low-fat spreads on bread and vegetables (Table 4.7(vii)). While about a third of men and women report using sunflower/olive oil margarines on bread and vegetables, most indicated that they use pure vegetable oils for frying (65% for men and 66% for women).

Table 4.7. Percentage distribution of respondents' frequency of food consumption by gender

(i) Bread[1]

	Less than 1 a day		1–2 a day		3–4 a day		5 or more a day		Totals	
	M (%)	W (%)[2]	M (%)	W (%)	M (%)	W (%)	M (%)	W (%)	M (%)	W (%)
White bread	2	3	11	19	20	19*	23	5	56	45
Brown or granary bread	1	2	4	12	8	9*	7	3	20	25
Wholemeal bread	1	2*	6	13	10	12	18	3	24	29
Never eat bread									1	2
Base:[3]									2 730	2 782

[1]Q163 About how many pieces of bread or rolls do you eat on a usual day? Are they usually white, brown or wholemeal?
[2]Chi-squared test for differences between men and women statistically significant p < 0.05 unless marked *
[3]Base: missing 1% men and 1% women

(ii) Breakfast cereals[1]

	Less than 1 a day		1–2 a day		3–4 a day		5 or more a day		Totals	
	M (%)	W (%)[2]	M (%)	W (%)	M (%)	W (%)	M (%)	W (%)	M (%)	W (%)
Sugar types	<1	1	2	1	1	1*	2	1	6	4
Rice/corn	2	2*	7	6*	8	6	11	10*	28	23
Porridge	1	1*	1	1†	1	2	3	2	6	6*
Wheat	1	1*	3	4*	4	6	12	9	20	19*
Muesli	<1	1*	1	2	3	2*	4	4*	8	9*
Bran	1	1*	1	2	2	4	5	8	9	15
Never eat breakfast cereals									25	25
Base:[3]									2 741	2 785

[1]Q164 About how many times a week do you have a bowl of cereal or porridge? What kind do you have most often?
[2]Chi-squared test for differences between men and women statistically significant p < 0.05 unless marked *
[3]Base: < 1% missing men and 1% missing women
†Actual figures 1.2% and 0.6% for men and women respectively

(iii) Starchy foods and fruit and vegetables[1]

	Less than 1 a week		1–2 a week		3–5 a week		6 or more a week	
	M (%)	W (%)[2]	M (%)	W (%)	M (%)	W (%)	M (%)	W (%)
Rice, spaghetti or noodles	29	30*	53	53*	16	16*	2	2*
Potatoes	2	4	18	21	50	48*	30	27
Peas	15	22	49	51*	31	24	5	4
Baked beans, dried beans or lentils	25	32	55	52*	17	15*	3	1
Other vegetables (any type)	3	2*	15	12	39	32	43	54
Fruit (fresh, frozen or canned)	13	8	22	14	23	20	42	59

Base:[3]

[1]Q165 About how many times a week do you eat the following foods?
[2]Chi-squared test for differences between men and women statistically significant p < 0.05 unless marked *
[3]Base: missing 1% men and 1% women

(iv) Meat[1]

	Less than 1 a week		1–2 a week		3–5 a week		6 or more a week	
	M (%)	W (%)[2]	M (%)	W (%)	M (%)	W (%)	M (%)	W (%)
Beefburgers/sausages	45	63	47	35	6	2	1	<1
Beef/pork/lamb	20	26	57	56*	20	17	2	2*
Bacon/meat pies/pasties	30	42	53	49	14	8	3	1
Chicken/turkey	20	17	64	63*	16	20	1	1*
Fish (not fried)	46	40	46	50	7	10	1	1*

Base:[3]

[1]Q166 About how many times a week do you eat a serving of the following foods?
[2]Chi-squared test for differences between men and women statistically significant p < 0.05 unless marked *
[3]Base: missing 1% men and 1% women

(v) Cheese, fried foods, cakes and biscuits[1]

	Less than 1 a week		1–2 a week		3–5 a week		6 or more a week	
	M (%)	W (%)[2]	M (%)	W (%)	M (%)	W (%)	M (%)	W (%)
Cheese (except cottage)	19	22	37	35 *	32	30 *	13	13 *
Any fried food	34	50	45	42	18	8	4	1
Cakes/pies/puddings	29	31 *	37	36 *	20	21 *	15	12
Biscuits/chocolates	19	23	25	25 *	24	24 *	32	29
Base:[3]								

[1]Q167 About how many times a week do you eat a serving of the following foods?
[2]Chi-squared test for differences between men and women statistically significant p < 0.05 unless marked *
[3]Base: missing 1% men and 1% women

(vi) Milk[1]

	Less than $\frac{1}{4}$ pint		About $\frac{1}{4}$ pint		About $\frac{1}{2}$ pint		1 pint or more		Total	
	M (%)	W (%)[2]	M (%)	W (%)	M (%)	W (%)	M (%)	W (%)	M (%)	W (%)
Full cream milk	3	3 *	4	4 *	14	13 *	17	9	37	28
Semi-skimmed milk	2	5	5	7	20	24	20	13	48	50
Skimmed milk	1	2 *	2	2 *	5	8	4	5	12	18
Never use milk									3	4
Base:[3]									2 730	2 780

[1]Q168 About how much milk do you yourself use in a day, for drinking or in cereal, tea or coffee? What kind of milk do you usually use? 3% men and 4% women never use milk
[2]Chi-squared test for differences between men and women statistically significant p < 0.05 unless marked *
[3]Base: missing 1% men and 1% women

(vii) Sort of fat used for spread on bread, frying and baking[1]

	Fat used on bread and vegetables		Fat used for frying		Fat used for baking or cooking	
	M (%)	W (%)[2]	M (%)	W (%)	M (%)	W (%)
Butter/ghee/dripping	23	20	13	13 *	18	17 *
Hard/soft margarine	17	14	3	3 *	21	32
Sunflower/olive margarine	35	33 *	5	5 *	13	19
Low-fat spreads	21	29	1	1 *	3	4 *
Pure vegetable oils	1	1 *	65	66 *	21	15
None	3	4 *	13	12 *	26	13
Base:[3]	2 744	2 787	2 714	2 775	2 658	2 766

[1]Q169 to Q171 What sort of fat do you use on bread, for frying, for baking? Single code only
[2]Chi-squared test for differences between men and women statistically significant p < 0.05 unless marked *
[3]Base: missing <1% men and <1% women Q169; 1% men and 1% women Q170, 3% men and 1% women Q171

The food consumption patterns reported in the present survey were similar to those recently reported in the Health Survey for England (Bennett *et al.*, 1995), the National Food Survey (1994) and an earlier national consumption study (Gregory *et al.*, 1990).

The percentage of subjects with DINE scores for fat, unsaturated fat, fibre and fruit and vegetables broken down into lowest, moderate and highest intake categories is presented in Table 4.8. Men are more likely than women to be in the lowest consumption category for unsaturated fat and fruit and vegetables, and in the highest consumption categories for fat and fibre. The gender differences for fat were to be expected given that men eat absolutely more food, and therefore fat; if the fat distribution had been expressed relative to energy intake the gender differences would have been much smaller. Over 60% of women are in the highest category of fruit consumption.

Within each gender group more younger subjects were in the highest fat group (for example, 54% of 16- to 19-year-old men compared with 28% in 55- to 64-year-old men). Male current smokers were also more likely to be in the highest fat group (48% among current smokers compared with 33% in never smokers). Regional differences in the percentage of subjects in the highest fat index group were apparent; for males the greatest contrast was between West Midlands (46%) and North Thames (31%); for females the contrast was between the North West (23%) and South and West and North Thames (12%). All of the comparisons mentioned above were statistically significant.

The demographic characteristics of subjects in the low fruit and vegetable group were explored further. Younger women (16% compared to the oldest age group 7%) and men (23% compared with 10% in the oldest group) were more likely to be in the low consumption category, as were smokers

Table 4.8. Percentage distribution of respondents' food intake scores from the DINE questionnaire by gender[1]

	Low		Moderate		High	
	M (%)	W (%)[2]	M (%)	W (%)	M (%)	W (%)
Fat	30	50	34	32*	37	18
Unsaturated fat	10	9	37	38*	53	54*
Fibre	34	44	38	35	28	21
Fruit and vegetables	15	10	40	28	45	62
Base:[3]						

[1]Q163 to Q172
[2]Chi-squared test for differences between men and women statistically significant p < 0.05 unless marked *
[3]Base: number (and % missing) for men and women respectively:
 Fat 2646 (4%) and 2711 (3%);
 Unsaturated fat 2650 (4%) and 2759 (1%);
 Fibre 2695 (2%) and 2749 (2%);
 Fruit and vegetables 2740 (1%) and 2782 (1%)

Table 4.9. Percentage distribution of dietary cluster variable computed from food frequencies by gender[1]

	Men (%)	Women (%)[2]
Less healthy diet	53	43
More healthy diet	47	57
Base:[3]	2 669	2 716

[1]Q163 to Q171
[2]Chi-squared test for differences between men and women statistically significant p < 0.05
[3]Base: missing 3% men and 3% women

compared with never smokers (for men 20% compared with 12%). Female respondents on income support were more likely to be in the low fruit and vegetable consumption group compared with women not on income support (24% compared with 8%). The greatest regional contrasts were between South Thames and North West (6% compared with 13%) for women, and between Anglia and Oxford and West Midlands (11% compared with 19%) for men. All of the above comparisons were statistically significant.

For most of the demographic questions asked there were differences in the percentage of subjects reporting a high-fat diet and a low fruit-vegetable diet. To simplify interpretation cluster analyses were used to derive two scores: one reflecting the respondents' overall socio-demographic profile (four levels); and one reflecting their diet (two levels). For simplicity the dietary clusters have been described as more and less 'healthy'. Table 4.9 presents the percentage of subjects in each cluster by gender. Fifty-three per cent of men and 43% of women were grouped into the less healthy cluster.

Comparing the dietary clusters with the demographic clusters, this shows that 64% of the cluster characterised as the younger, low-income families (cluster 2) were eating a diet defined as less healthy; this compares with 41% among subjects in the cluster defined as middle-aged educated (Figure 4.8).

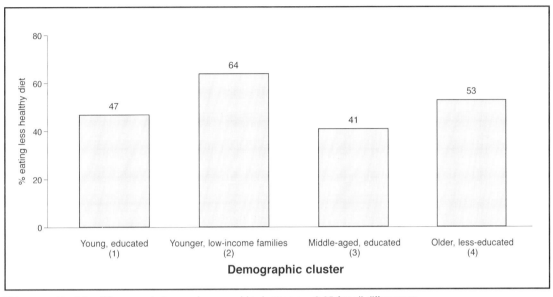

Chi-squared test for differences between demographic clusters p < 0.05 for all differences

Fig. 4.8. Percentage of respondents classified as eating a less healthy diet by demographic cluster

Dividing the regions into a simple North–South divide, 47% of women and 57% of men in the North were eating a less healthy diet compared with 40% of women and 49% for men in the South (the difference was statistically significant).

Eating patterns

Subjects were asked questions about their usual eating arrangements, such as where they ate meals and with whom (Tables 4.10 and 4.11). Thirty per cent of men and 26% of women normally eat their meals in the living room in front of the television; about half of the respondents either eat their meals in the kitchen or dining room at the table.

Younger men and women were more likely to eat their meals watching television. The overwhelming majority (95%) of respondents said that they had a meal or snack with all or most other members of their family; about two-thirds of the respondents said they did this at least every day (Table 4.11).

Table 4.10. Percentage distribution of the room in which meals are normally eaten by gender[1]

	Men (%)	Women (%)[2]
Living room at a table	15	15
Living room, in front of television	30	26 †
Dining room, at a table	27	28
Kitchen	24	27 †
It depends	2	2
Never eat at home	0	0
Other	2	1
Base:[3]	2 746	2 793

[1]Q125 Which room do you normally eat your meals in?
[2]Chi-squared test for differences between men and women statistically significant p < 0.05 marked †
[3]Base: missing <1% men and <1% women

Table 4.11. Percentage distribution of the frequency of eating meals with other members of the household by gender[1]

	Men (%)	Women (%)[2]
Two/three times a day	25	28 †
Once a day	49	48
Every 2–3 days	12	10
Every 4–5 days	9	7 †
Once a week	4	5
Less than once a week	1	1
Don't know/no answer	<1	<1
Base:[3]	2 388	2 440

[1]Q140 About how often would you say you do this?
[2]Chi-squared test for differences between men and women statistically significant p < 0.05 marked †
[3]Base: respondents who eat with other members of the household.

Eighty-three per cent of subjects who ate with their family, ate their evening meal with their family, and three-quarters said that they ate Sunday lunch with their family.

Subjects were also asked about eating practices at lunch time (Table 4.12). Of those subjects who work and were not self-employed, 48% of men and 36% of women brought a packed lunch from home and 22% of men and 19% of women ate in a workplace canteen (not statistically significant). Men employed in manual occupations were more likely to eat a packed lunch from home than non-manual men (56% compared with 41%) whereas for women the reverse was the case (24% in manual women and 42% in non-manual women). For 22% of men and 17% of women, lunch was their main meal of the day during weekdays. All of the above comparisons were statistically significant unless indicated.

Table 4.12. Percentage distribution of the place where lunch is eaten whilst at work by gender[1]

	Men (%)	Women (%)[2]
Workplace canteen	22	19*
Pub	3	1
Cafe/take-away/sandwich bar	11	8
Restaurant	4	1
Shop	4	4*
Vending machine on-site	1	<1
Vending machine off-site	<1	0
Lunch supplied at meetings	<1	0*
Bring packed lunch from home	48	36
Often miss lunch/never have lunch	3	3*
Don't have lunch at work	4	12
Go home for lunch	6	12
Other	4	7
Don't know/no answer	1	3
Base:[3]	1 265	1 404

[1]Q143 When you are at work, where do you usually obtain lunch? Multiple response question
[2]Chi-squared test for differences between men and women statistically significant p < 0.05 unless marked *
[3]Base: respondents who work and are not self-employed

For respondents who did the shopping two-thirds used local supermarkets, about 30% used out-of-town supermarkets (Table 4.13). More than two-thirds of respondents go shopping in their cars, and about 20% walk, mainly to local shops. Virtually all respondents who shop in out-of-town supermarkets use their car (85% of men and 89% of women). Respondents with partners were more likely to use out of town supermarkets than those with no partner in the household (33% and 23% for men and women). When the place of shopping was broken down by demographic cluster the middle-aged educated cluster group was more likely to shop out of town than the younger, low-income families group (33% for cluster 3 compared with 19% for cluster 2) (Figure 4.9), probably explained by car ownership.

Table 4.13. Percentage distribution of places where most food is bought by the respondent by gender[1]

	Men (%)	Women (%)[2]
Small local shops	12	7 †
Local supermarkets	67	67
Supermarkets in other towns or other parts of towns	29	30
Markets	5	4
Food halls in department stores	<1	1
Farms and farm stalls	1	1
Mobile shops	<1	<1
Other	1	<1
Don't know/no answer	2	<1 †
Base:[3]	923	2 328

[1]Q102 Which one of the places on this list do you buy most of your food in? Multiple question
[2]Chi-squared test for differences between men and women statistically significant p < 0.05 when marked †
[3]Base: respondents who do most of the shopping

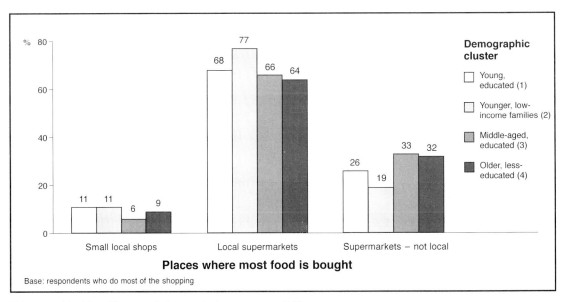

Base: respondents who do most of the shopping

Chi-squared test for differences between cluster groups p < 0.05:
Small local shops – cluster 3 different from other clusters
Local supermarkets – cluster 2 different from other clusters
Supermarkets not local – all except 3 versus 4

Fig. 4.9. Percentage distribution of places where most food is bought by demographic cluster group

Table 4.14 describes the reasons people gave for shopping where they did. Convenience was the most commonly mentioned factor followed by price. Only 8% of respondents mentioned a good range of healthy choices as a factor. When reasons for shopping were broken down by demographic cluster group (Figure 4.10) for all groups, except cluster 2, convenience was the most commonly mentioned reason affecting place of shopping. The biggest contrast was for affordability between clusters 2 (younger, low-income families) and 3 (middle-aged educated) (52% compared with 25%).

Table 4.14. Percentage distribution of reasons for choice of place where respondents do most of their shopping by gender[1]

	Men (%)	Women (%)[2]
Prices are affordable	38	31
Good range of healthy choices	9	8
Good quality food	11	10
Quick or convenient to get to	59	58
Foods are fresh	5	6
Wide range of foods available	20	21
Shop/outlet is clean	1	2†
Sell things other than foods/can do all shopping in same place	14	16
My family or friends go there	1	1
I've always done my shopping there	5	4
Other[3]	9	12†
Don't know/no answer	1	<1
Base:[4]	906	2 322

[1]Q103 And why do you do most of your shopping in .... ? Multiple response questions
[2]Chi-squared test for differences between men and women statistically significant p < 0.05 when marked †
[3]Includes good parking, good staff, no choice, like to support local shops
[4]Base: respondents who shop and named place where shop

When subjects were asked what factors they thought about when they go shopping, cost was the single most important factor, more so for women than men (52% compared with 43%) (Table 4.15). The third most common answer was trying to eat a healthy diet (22% for men and 23% for women). Advertising seemed to have little influence. Younger men and women were more likely to be influenced by cost than older respondents (48% for young men compared with 40% for older men; 64% for younger women compared with 46% in older women). Trends across age groups were statistically significant in women but not men. When food buying choices were broken down by the demographic cluster variable, cost was still the main factor for all cluster groups, but more so for younger, low-income families (cluster 2) (Figure 4.11).

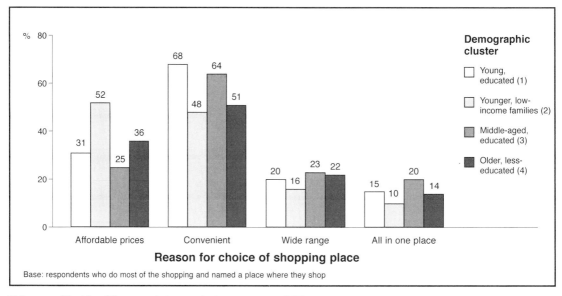

Chi-squared test for differences between cluster groups p < 0.05
Affordable prices – all; Convenient – all except 2 v. 4, 1 v. 3; Wide range – 2 v. 3 different only
All in one place – 3 compared with other clusters, 1 v. 2, 2 v. 4

Fig. 4.10. Percentage distribution of reasons for choice of place where most of the shopping is bought by demographic cluster group

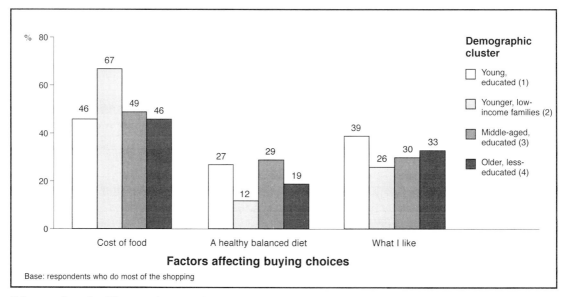

Chi-squared test for differences between clusters p < 0.05
Cost of food – 2 different from other clusters; A healthy balanced diet – all differences except 1 v. 3;
What I like – all differences except 2 v. 3, 3 v. 4

Fig. 4.11. Percentage distribution of reasons affecting food buying choices by demographic cluster group

Table 4.15. Percentage of subjects indicating various factors affecting choice of foods when shopping by gender[1]

	Men (%)	Women (%)[2]
Cost of foods/my food budget	43	52 †
Prescribed diet	4	4
What spouse/partner will eat	8	14 †
What my child/children will eat	6	13 †
Trying to eat a healthy balanced diet	22	23
The kind of foods I like eating	37	31 †
Convenience	9	9
Whether my spouse/partner is with me	1	1
Whether my child/children are with me	<1	1 †
Packaging/display	4	6
Food advertising	1	1
Items/programmes in media	1	1
The kind of foods my friends buy	<1	<1
The kind of foods my relatives buy	1	<1
Whether I'm hungry or not	1	1
Religious/cultural reasons	1	<1
Vegetarian/vegan	3	4
Other[3]	27	26
Don't know/no answer	6	5
Base:[4]	923	2 328

[1]Q106 When you go food shopping, what factors do you think affect the choice of foods you buy? Multiple question
[2]Chi-squared test for differences between men and women statistically significant (p < 0.05 when marked †
[3]Includes quality, freshness, variety, special offers, only buy what I need, ingredients/additives
[4]Base: all respondents who do most of the shopping

Body mass index

Based on self-reported data:

- A third of women aged 16–19 years are underweight.

- Fourteen per cent of men and women aged 45–54 years are obese.

- More manual workers are obese than non-manual workers.

Subjects were asked their height and weight, and body mass index (weight over height squared) was calculated. Previous research has shown that both perceived height and weight are likely to be reasonable proxy measures for true weight and height (Stunkard and Albaum, 1981), although they may be misleading for the obese (Kuskowska-Wolk *et al.*, 1989). Body mass index was divided into four broad groupings: underweight (less than 20 kg/m²), average (20 up to 25), overweight (25–30) and obese (over 30) and Table 4.16 presents the percentage of subjects in each category broken down by gender. Most men and women fall within the average or overweight categories; women were more likely to be underweight than men (9% for women compared with 4% for men). The prevalences of underweight and obesity reported here are similar to that reported previously (Gregory *et al.*, 1990).

Table 4.16. Percentage distribution of body mass index into various categories by gender[1]

	Men (%)	Women (%)[2]
Underweight (BMI = 20 or less kg/m²)	4	9
Average (BMI = 20.1–25.0 kg/m²)	45	50
Overweight (BMI = 25.1–29.9 kg/m²)	40	29
Obese (BMI = 30 or more kg/m²)	11	12
Base:[3]	2 716	2 697

[1]Q90 and Q91: Self-reported height and weight
[2]Chi-squared test for differences between men and women statistically significant $p < 0.05$ unless marked *
[3]Base: missing 1% men and 4% women

Thirty-one per cent of women aged 16 to 19 years of age were defined as underweight, whereas only about 4% of women over 45 years of age were underweight. The comparison for men was 22% and 3%, for 16- to 19-year-olds compared with men over 45 years of age. By contrast less than 5% of young men and women were obese compared with over 14% of men and women aged 45 to 54 years of age. The prevalence of obesity was higher in manual workers than non-manual workers (men – non-manual 8%, manual 13%; women – non-manual 11%, manual 17%). The prevalence of obesity was highest in men in the Northern Yorkshire and West Midlands regions (13%) and lowest in the North West region (8%). For women, the prevalence of obesity was highest in the Northern, Yorkshire and Trent regions (16%) and lowest in the Anglia and Oxford region (9%). Using the demographic cluster variable to summarise the demographic variables showed that the prevalence of obesity was 5.5% in cluster 1 (young, educated) and 15% in cluster 4 (older, less-educated); this contrast is most strongly affected by age, with young single persons in cluster 1 and older married couples in cluster 4.

Current smokers were least likely to be obese compared with ex-smokers (men – current 10%, ex- 13%; women – current 10%, ex- 16%). Female smokers were also more likely to be underweight than ex-smokers (13% compared with 6% underweight in current and ex-smokers respectively). For male respondents but not females those in the obese group (71%) were more likely to believe people could reduce their risk of heart disease by controlling bodyweight than those in the underweight group (55%).

Barriers to change

This section explores attitudes towards healthy eating and the types of changes people have made to their diets over the last three years. The reasons why changes had or had not been made, and the barriers to change are discussed.

- About one-third of men and women are confused about healthy eating.

- Respondents that ate a healthy diet were more likely to think that fresh fruit and vegetables were part of a healthy diet, and that eating more fruit and vegetables could reduce people's risk of heart disease.

- Many people have changed their diets over the last three years, although younger people in manual occupations have made least change.

- Demographic profile was a strong determinant of eating patterns, perceptions about a healthy diet and barriers to change to a healthy diet. The younger, low-income families and older less-educated groups were less likely to eat a healthy diet or to have changed their diets, more likely to believe that healthy diets are a fashion and expensive, and to have cost as a limiting factor in where to shop and what to buy.

Attitudes

Respondents were asked to indicate their level of agreement with a series of statements about eating (Table 4.17(i)–(iii)). The majority of men and women disagreed with the statements that healthy eating was just another fashion, and that they don't really care what they eat. About a third of men and women agreed with the statement that they get confused over what is supposed to be healthy and what is not; about 40% of men and women agreed that eating healthy foods was expensive. Women were slightly more likely than men to agree with the statement that feeding their family what they like is more important than trying to eat healthy foods (30% compared with 22%).

Older men and women were more likely than younger men and women to agree that healthy eating was just another fashion (older women – 20% compared with 9% for younger women; for men – 23% compared with 16%).

Young men (under 25 years of age) compared with older men and women of all ages were more likely to agree with the statement that they don't care what they eat (27% compared with 19% in young and older respectively).

For most statements there were differences in the way respondents in manual and non-manual occupational groups answered (Table 4.18). Men and women in manual occupations were more likely to agree that eating more healthy foods was just a fashion (men 25% compared with 14% for manual and non-manual respectively and for women 19% compared with 13%). Both men and women in manual occupations compared with those in non-manual occupations were more likely to agree that eating more healthy foods was expensive (men – manual 46%, non-manual 29%; women – manual 48%, non-manual 36%). Men and women in manual occupations were also more likely to agree that they get confused over what is supposed to be a healthy diet (men – 47% and 30% for manual and non-manual men respectively and for women 40% and 26%) and more likely to agree that feeding their family what they like is more important than trying to eat healthy foods (for men 32% compared with 13%; for women 39% compared with 22%).

Responses were also broken down by the demographic cluster variable to provide a simpler overall summary of the effect of these demographic factors (Figure 4.12(i)–(v)). The middle-aged educated demographic cluster (cluster 3) were the group least likely to agree that healthy eating was just another fashion, or that they don't care about what they eat, or get confused over what was supposed to be healthy. For expense and don't care the greatest contrast with cluster group 2 (younger, low-income families) was either cluster 1 or cluster 3. (Expense cluster 2, 56%, cluster 1, 32%, cluster 3, 33%; don't care cluster 2, 27%, cluster 3, 11%). Younger, low-income family respondents were also more likely to agree with the statement that their partner persuades them to buy unhealthy foods, and feeding their family what they like was more important than trying to eat healthy foods.

Table 4.17. Percentage distribution of barriers to healthy eating/dietary change by gender[1]

(i)	% Strongly agree		% Tend to agree		% Neither agree or disagree		% Tend to disagree		% Strongly disagree		% Don't know/no answer	
	M	W[2]	M	W	M	W	M	W	M	W	M	W
Healthy eating is just another fashion[3]	4	3*	16	13	7	6	36	38*	35	39	3	2
It's not very easy to eat healthy foods if you eat out	8	7*	30	25	10	10*	33	39	11	14	9	7
Eating healthy food is expensive	11	11*	27	29*	11	9	35	37*	11	12*	6	2
Healthy foods are enjoyable	21	27	52	54*	16	11	8	6	2	1*	2	2*
The tastiest foods are the ones that are bad for you	20	22	31	29*	12	10*	25	27*	10	11*	3	2

(i) cont'd	% Strongly agree		% Tend to agree		% Neither agree or disagree		% Tend to disagree		% Strongly disagree		% Don't know/no answer	
	M	W[2]	M	W	M	W	M	W	M	W	M	W
I don't really care what I eat	7	3	14	8	7	5	33	37	38	47	1	1 *
I get confused over what's supposed to be healthy and what isn't	8	6	31	26	8	6	32	36	19	24	2	1 *
Experts never agree about what foods are good for you	25	24 *	46	48 *	11	9 *	12	13 *	3	3 *	4	3 *

[1]Q111 How strongly do you agree or disagree with the following statements?
[2]Chi-squared test for differences between men and women statistically significant $p < 0.05$ unless marked *
[3]Base: 2334 men and 3219 women

(ii)	% Strongly agree		% Tend to agree		% Neither agree or disagree		% Tend to disagree		% Strongly disagree		% Don't know/no answer	
	M	W[1]	M	W	M	W	M	W	M	W	M	W
My partner always wants to eat the foods he/she is familiar with[1]	10	21	31	29 *	7	4	34	31	16	15 *	1	1 *
My partner often persuades me to buy unhealthy foods[2]	2	6	6	13	4	5	38	39 *	49	35	2	1

[1]Chi-squared test for differences between men and women statistically significant $p < 0.05$ unless marked *
[2]Base: those who live with partner: 1804 men and 1908 women

(iii)	% Strongly agree		% Tend to agree		% Neither agree or disagree		% Tend to disagree		% Strongly disagree		% Don't know/no answer	
	M	W[1]	M	W	M	W	M	W	M	W	M	W
Feeding my family what they like is more important than trying to eat healthy foods[1]	4	7	18	23	14	14 *	40	36 *	21	18 *	3	2 *
My child/ren always want to eat the foods they're familiar with	19	21 *	47	43 *	7	6 *	19	21 *	5	8	4	2
My children often persuade to buy unhealthy foods[2]	6	13	23	27 *	13	8	32	30 *	21	19 *	5	3 *

[1]Chi-squared test for differences between men and women statistically significant $p < 0.05$ unless marked *
[2]Base: parents with children in household: 827 men and 943 women

Table 4.18. Percentage distribution of barriers to healthy eating/dietary change by occupational group by gender

	Agree (%)		Neither agree or disagree (%)		Disagree (%)	
	M	W	M	W	M	W
Healthy eating is just another fashion						
Non-manual[1,2]	14	13	5	5	81	81
Manual	25	19	9	6*	63	73
Eating healthy food is expensive						
Non-manual	29	36	10	9	58	53
Manual	46	48	11*	9*	35	42
I don't really care what I eat						
Non-manual	13	8	6	4	81	87
Manual	29	14	8	5*	63	79
I get confused over what's supposed to be healthy and what isn't						
Non-manual	30	26	8	6	61	67
Manual	47	40	7*	6*	44	53
Feeding my family what they like is more important than trying to eat healthy food[2]						
Non-manual	13	22	15	14	69	62
Manual	32	39	13*	14*	51	45

[1]Chi-squared test for differences between non-manual and manual groups by gender statistically significant $p < 0.05$ unless marked *
[2]Base: parents with children in household: 827 men and 943 women

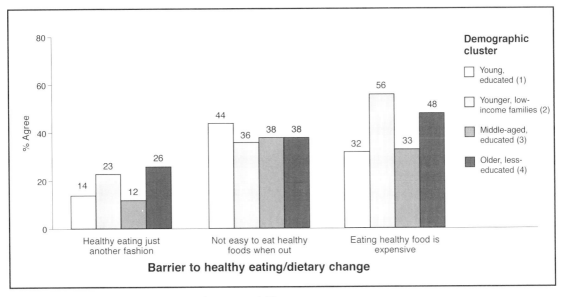

Chi-squared test for differences between clusters p < 0.05
Just another fashion – all except 1 v. 3, 2 v. 4; Not easy when eat out – all except 2 v. 3, 2 v. 4, 3 v. 4
Expensive – all except 1 v. 3

(i) Healthy eating is just another fashion, it's not easy to eat healthy foods when out, eating healthy food is expensive

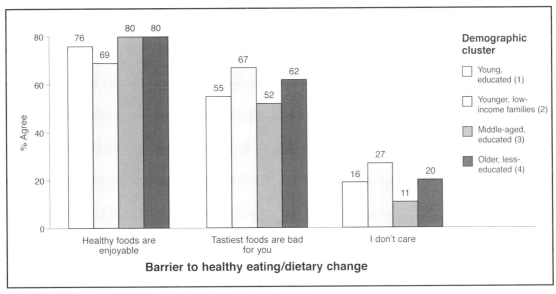

Chi-squared test for differences between clusters p < 0.05
Enjoyable – all except 3 v. 4; Tastiest foods are bad for you – all except 1 v. 3; I don't care – all

(ii) Healthy foods are enjoyable, tastiest foods are bad for you, I don't care

Fig. 4.12. Percentage agreeing with barriers to healthy eating/dietary change by demographic cluster group

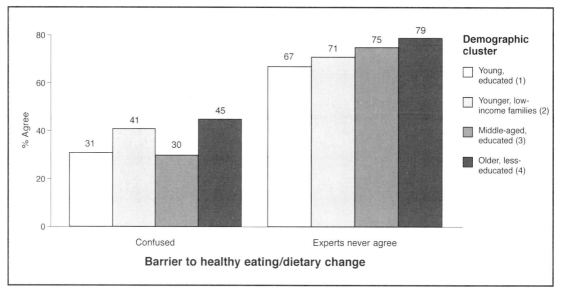

Chi-squared test for differences between clusters p < 0.05
Confused – all except 1 v. 3, 2 v. 4
Experts never agree – all except 2 v. 3, 1 v. 2

(iii) Confused over what's supposed to be healthy and what isn't, experts never agree about what foods are good for you

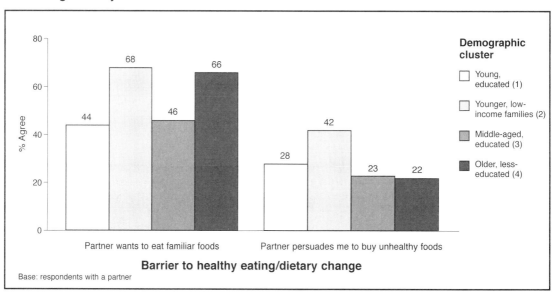

Chi-squared test for differences between clusters p < 0.05
Familiar foods – all except 1 v. 3, 2 v. 4
Unhealthy foods – all except 1 v. 3, 3 v. 4

(iv) Partner wants to eat familiar foods, partner persuades me to buy unhealthy foods

Fig. 4.12. Percentage agreeing with barriers to healthy eating/dietary change by demographic cluster group

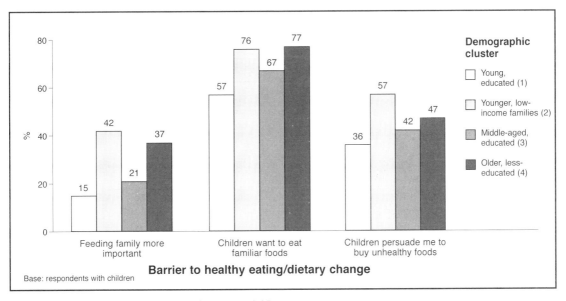

Chi-squared test for difference between clusters p < 0.05
Feeding the family – all except 1 v. 3, 2. v. 4
Familiar foods – all except 1 v. 3, 2 v. 4
Unhealthy foods – only 1 v. 2, 2 v. 3

(v) Feeding the family is more important, children want to eat familiar foods, children persuade me to buy unhealthy foods

Fig. 4.12. Percentage agreeing with barriers to healthy eating/dietary change by demographic cluster group

Behaviour

These contrasts highlight some obvious, but important differences which need to be addressed in the way health promotion programmes are developed. If achieving better health through changes in diet is the aim of health promotion in this area, then ultimately what is of greatest importance is not what people's knowledge and attitudes are, but what they actually do. Characterising differences between those who eat 'healthy' diets and those who do not will help target health promotion activity. It may be important to explore the willingness of people to change their diets and the constraints people feel on that change; some people will not see the need for change because they are, or feel they are, already eating a healthy diet.

Subjects were asked to describe a healthy diet; over 70% mentioned that a healthy diet includes fresh fruit and vegetables, 34% mentioned it should include high fibre cereals, 38% mentioned fish and white meat and 22% mentioned pasta and rice. Superficially these data suggest that the majority of people have a sense of what is currently recommended as being the basis of a healthy diet.

Subjects were then asked if they have changed their diet over the last three years (Table 4.19). Forty-nine per cent of men and 39% of women stated that

Table 4.19. Percentage distribution of the dietary changes respondents have made over the last three years by gender[1]

	Men (%)	Women (%)[2]
Eat less generally	5	5 *
Eat less convenience foods/fast foods/takeaways	4	3 *
Eat less fat	12	15
Eat less red meat/fatty meat	11	14
Eat less fried food	9	8 *
Eat less sugar/sweets/chocolates/biscuits/cakes	11	15
Eat less eggs	2	2 *
Drink less alcohol	3	2
Drink less whole milk	2	3 *
Drink less fizzy drinks	1	1 *
Switched to lower-fat food	4	6
Switched to lean meats	2	2 *
Switched to polyunsaturated/monounsaturated fats	4	6
Switched to low-fat spreads	3	5
Switched to skimmed/semi-skimmed milk	8	12
Eat more high-fibre food	7	10
Eat more starchy food	5	6 *
Eat more fruit/vegetables/salad	13	16
Eat more fish	4	4 *
Eat more lean meat	3	3 *
Change cooking methods	3	4 *
Other more healthy changes[3]	2	3
Other less healthy changes[4]	2	2 *
Other[5]	6	7 *
None (no changes)	49	39
Don't know/no answer	1	1 *
Base:	2 754	2 799

[1]Q113 In what ways, if any, have you changed your diet over the last three years? Multiple response question
[2]Chi-squared test for differences between men and women statistically significant p < 0.05 unless marked *
[3]Includes eat more white meat, eat more regularly, balance of diet, healthier diet generally
[4]Includes eat more convenience food, eat less starchy foods, eat less fruit/vegetables/salad, eat more fat/sugary foods
[5]Includes – become vegetarian, eat less/more dairy food, eat more foreign food
In addition <1% men or women answered join a slimming club, go to see doctor or dietitian, take vitamin supplements, take other food supplement or buy meal replacements

Table 4.20. Percentage distribution of reasons given by respondents for no dietary changes in last three years by gender[1]

	Men (%)	Women (%)[2]
Already eating a healthy diet	52	60
Not interested/cannot be bothered/don't believe it's important for me	12	8
None of the experts seem to agree, so why should I change?	7	4
I don't know enough about which foods are good for you	10	5
It's expensive	4	5 *
Pressure/resistance to change from spouse/partner	2	2 *
Pressure/resistance to change from children	1	2
I don't really believe the food you eat affects your health	2	1 *
Not enough time to cook/prepare/buy healthy foods	5	6 *
I don't need to worry about the food I eat at my age	7	4
I like the taste of the food that I already eat	23	20 *
I take plenty of exercise therefore I can eat what I like	6	3
Now I have less money to spend on food	5	5 *
I wouldn't enjoy eating healthier foods	3	2 *
Travel/moving around	3	1
Difficult to get access to cooking facilities	1	1 *
Family upset/disruption	1	2 *
Other responsibilities mean I don't have time to cook for myself	4	3 *
Other	3	4 *
Don't know/no answer	3	4 *
Base:[3]	1 347	1 101

[1]Q116 Which of these best describes your reasons for not having made an effort to eat a healthy diet over the last three years? Multiple response question

[2]Chi-squared test for differences between men and women statistically significant $p < 0.05$ unless marked *

[3]Base: respondents who replied 'none' at Q113

they had made no change in their diet. The most commonly mentioned dietary changes were to eat more fruit and vegetables (13% for men and 16% for women), eat less fat (12% men, 15% women) and eat less sugar and sweets (11% men, 15% women).

Those respondents who indicated that they had not changed their diets were asked which of a list of reasons best described why they had made no change (Table 4.20). Over half of those subjects who made no change had done so because they were already eating a healthy diet. The next most common answer was because 'I like the taste of the food that I already eat' (23% for men and 20% for women). Few subjects mentioned expense.

Table 4.21. Percentage distribution of respondents' dietary changes in last three years by gender[1]

	Men (%)	Women (%)
No dietary changes various reasons[2]	24 [7]	16
No dietary changes, diet already healthy[3]	26	24 *
Other changes[4]	9	12
Made more healthy dietary changes[5]	47	57
Base:[6]	2 727	2 775

[1] Chi-squared test for differences between men and women statistically significant p < 0.05 unless marked *
[2] Q113 no changes and Q116 all reasons except diet already healthy
[3] Q113 no changes and Q116 diet already healthy
[4] Q113 other changes and less healthy changes
[5] Q113 changes eat less generally to join a slimming class
[6] Base: Missing 1% men and 1% women
[7] Percentages do not add up to 100% as some respondents made other dietary changes as well as more healthy dietary changes

Combining the data from Tables 4.19 and 4.20 for all subjects showed that 47% of men and 57% of women have reported making dietary changes in the last three years, and about a quarter stated that they were already eating a healthy diet (Table 4.21).

The summary change data presented in Table 4.21 were broken down by the various demographic variables and finally the demographic cluster variable. Younger men (particularly) and women were the least likely to have changed their diets in the past three years (for men 34% no change in the younger group (16–24) compared with 20% in the older 45–74 age group). Men and women in manual occupations were also more likely not to have changed their diets (17% for non-manual compared with 29% for manual men; 12% for non-manual compared with 21% for manual women). All these comparisons were statistically significant. From the demographic cluster analysis the greatest contrast was between the younger low-income families cluster and the middle-aged educated cluster with 35% in the worst-off group making no changes compared with 13% in the better-off group.

The relationship between whether subjects had changed their diet and their responses to the various statements about diet suggested that those people who had not changed were more likely to agree that healthy eating is just a fashion compared with those who had changed their diets in the last three years (30% compared with 12% for women and 34% and 13% for men) (Table 4.22). Forty-five per cent of men and 27% of women who had not changed their diet in the last three years agreed that they didn't care about what they eat compared with 13% and 7% respectively for men and women who had changed their diets in the last three years. Overall these data suggest that

Table 4.22. Percentage distribution of agreement with barriers to healthy eating by dietary change in the last three years by gender

Barrier to dietary change	Men (%)		Women (%)	
	More healthy changes[1]	No change – various reasons	More healthy changes	No change – various reasons
Healthy eating is just another fashion	13	34	12	30
It's not very easy to eat healthy foods if you eat out	47	41	38	35 *
Eating healthy food is expensive	35	50	40	53
Healthy foods are enjoyable	77	57	83	63
The tastiest foods are the ones that are bad for you	58	64	58	69
I don't really care what I eat	13	45	7	27
I get confused over what's supposed to be healthy and what isn't	36	54	31	49
Experts never agree about what foods are good for you	74	76 *	73	77 *

[1]Chi-squared test for differences between more healthy changes and no change, various reasons statistically significant p < 0.05 unless marked *

those people who have not changed their diets are most likely to agree with potential reasons for not changing their diets.

Responses for dietary change were compared for subjects defined from the dietary cluster analysis to have a more or less healthy diet (Table 4.23). Over half (65% for women and 57% for men) of the respondents who had made changes to their diet were now eating diets which from the cluster analysis were defined as more healthy. In contrast, for both men and women, those who had not changed their diets were currently more likely to be consuming diets which were less healthy (men 75%; women 72%). For those who stated that they already had healthy diets, there was virtually no difference between the percentage of subjects eating a more or less healthy diet. Without objectively knowing what subjects ate in the past it must be assumed that those people who have changed their diets have done so for the better, but there is a proportion of those who believe they have changed to a healthy diet but are not currently eating the most healthy diets within the study population.

Table 4.23. Percentage distribution of dietary change in the last three years by dietary cluster by gender

Dietary change in last 3 years	Men (%)		Women (%)	
	Less healthy[1]	More healthy	Less healthy	More healthy
No change	75	25	72	28
Already healthy	48	52	42	58
Other changes	47	53	37	63
Change to more healthy diet	43	57	35	65

[1]Chi-squared test for differences between less healthy and more healthy diets all statistically significant p < 0.05

The relationship between people's perceptions of a healthy diet and their own diet was explored further. Respondents defined as having a more healthy diet from the dietary cluster analysis were more likely to agree with the statement that they mostly eat a healthy diet nowadays (more healthy diet cluster 85%, less healthy cluster 65%). For those subjects who mentioned that both fresh fruit and vegetables should be part of a healthy diet, 56% were eating a more healthy diet compared with 47% among those who did not mention either fruit or vegetables as part of a healthy diet. Among subjects in the middle-aged educated demographic cluster, about 60% of those who thought fresh fruit and vegetables were part of a healthy diet were eating a more healthy diet; whereas for the younger, low-income families only about 40% of those who mentioned fruit and vegetables as a healthy diet were eating a healthy diet.

Discussion

There are clear demographic differences which influence people's knowledge, attitudes and behaviour about nutrition. Programmes aimed at achieving dietary goals for healthy eating must recognise the underlying social, economic and demographic issues affecting people's knowledge and attitudes about access to a healthy diet if they are likely to succeed. Programmes need to be tailored more effectively to the needs of those groups most at risk. Many people from all socio-demographic groups are eating less healthy diets, but two-thirds of younger, low-income families are eating less healthy diets as defined by the cluster analysis. Cost was a major factor in influencing where people shop for food and what they buy, particularly among poorer groups.

Health promotion interventions aimed at improving health in the workplace through improving access to healthy foods in canteens (supported by such initiatives as the Heartbeat Award and Health at Work) may be missing some target groups. Whilst women in manual occupations are more likely to eat lunch from a workplace canteen than their non-manual counterparts, the same was not seen to be true for men. Most male manual workers eat a packed lunch from home. As only approximately one-fifth of respondents ate their midday meal in a workplace canteen the relative importance of workplace meals in the total diet needs to be taken into consideration in the planning of healthy eating interventions.

The responses to questions about fat revealed considerable inconsistency and confusion. People were asked questions about their own perceived confidence in explaining about fats and other foods. The accuracy of their perceptions was checked by asking them to identify foods high in fat. There is particular confusion over the fat content of margarine demonstrating the impact on people's health perceptions of commercial advertising. Many people thought wrongly that margarine was low in fat, clearly not distinguishing it from low-fat spreads. Conversely information levels were high and accurate about cholesterol. The less educated, and those in non-manual occupations had the poorest levels of knowledge.

There is also some indication within the data of needs for particular health education messages to be directed at the whole population to improve knowledge levels and reduce confusion about healthy eating. The final report of the Nutrition Task Force (Department of Health, 1996a), proposed the development of a common approach to the presentation to the public of the required balance of food in the diet. A schematic model for a food selection guide, graphical labelling, and a meal selection scheme were suggested. The HEA has produced the *National Food Guide: the balance of good health* to help people understand what is meant by a balanced diet. The approach emphasises the notion of balance, with selection of foods from broad food groups.

The task force recommended that a project team be established to analyse the possibilities to increase bread, pasta, rice and other cereal products, potatoes, fruit and vegetables and fish to replace reductions in fat. The task force recommended that gaps in knowledge about effective dietary interventions should be identified and the mechanisms developed to encourage research and development of effective interventions by the NHS.

The Nutrition Task Force, together with the Physical Activity Task Force (which reported in October 1995), proposed that attention should be directed towards prevention of obesity rather than its treatment. The prevalence of obesity has increased from 6% for men and 8% for women in 1980 to 13% for men and 16% for women in 1993. The Physical Activity Task Force also recommended targeted measures for those at greatest increase and new therapeutic strategies to help those who are already obese.

The report of the low-income Project Team (Department of Health, 1996b) identified the links between diet health and income; outlined numerous examples of local initiatives to improve the nutrition of low-income groups, and suggested further work to collate and disseminate examples of good practice.

While it appeared that respondents had reasonable knowledge about the important risk factors for CHD, the same could not be said for risk factors for diabetes, stroke and osteoporosis. Few people, for example, mentioned the benefits of exercise for reducing the risk of osteoporosis. Given the links between activity, energy expenditure, obesity and risk of chronic disease, a more integrated approach to promoting the benefits of physical activity could be important.

References

Bennett, N, Dodd, T, Flatley, J, Freeth, S and Bolling, K (1995). *Health survey for England 1993*. London: HMSO.

Department of Health (1995). *Obesity: reversing the increasing problem of obesity in England*. London: Department of Health.

Department of Health (1996a). *Eat Well II: a progress report from the Nutrition Task Force on the action plan to achieve the Health of the Nation targets on diet and nutrition*. London: Department of Health.

Department of Health (1996b). *Low income, food, nutrition and health: strategies for improvement: A report by the Low Income Project Team for the Department of Health Nutrition Task Force*. London: Department of Health.

Gregory, J, Foster, K, Tyler, H and Wiseman, M (1990). *The dietary and nutritional survey of British adults*. London: HMSO.

Holland, B, Welch, A A, Unwin, I D, Buss, D H, Paul, A A and Southgate, D A T (1991). *McCance and Widdowson's 'The Composition of Foods'*. 5th edn. London: Royal Society of Chemistry.

Kuskowska-Wolk, A, Karlsson, P, Stolt, M and Rössner, S (1989). The predictive validity of body mass index based on self-reported weight and height. *International Journal of Obesity* 13:441–53.

National Food Survey (1994). *Annual report on household food consumption and expenditure*. London: HMSO.

Roe, L, Strong, C, Whiteside, C, Neil, A and Mant, D (1994). Dietary intervention in primary care: validity of the DINE method for dietary assessment. *Family Practice* 11:375–81.

Stunkard, A J and Albaum, J M (1981). The accuracy of self-reported weights. *American Journal of Clinical Nutrition* 34:1593–9.

5. Sexual health

Introduction

This part of the report is restricted to respondents 16–54 years of age. Respondents completed the questionnaire themselves and answers were not checked. The response rate for this part of the questionnaire was 84%. This chapter has been divided into four sections: sexual behaviour; knowledge and attributes; contraception and condom use; and personal perceptions and risks of HIV.

Sexual behaviour

This section looks at age at first sexual intercourse and sexual partners in the last year in terms of numbers and type of relationships.

- Age at first intercourse is decreasing for both young men and women.

- Men and women in manual occupations are more likely to have their first intercourse under 16 years of age.

- Respondents in the poorer demographic cluster (A) are more likely to have had 2 or more partners in the last year.

- Men and women in 'steady' relationships are more likely to have had 2 or more partners in the last year than those married or living together.

Age at first sexual intercourse

Respondents were asked how old they were when they first had sexual intercourse (Table 5.1). Men were more likely to have first had sexual intercourse earlier than women; 43% of men having first had sex at 16 years of age or under compared with 32% for women; these differences were statistically significant.

Age at first intercourse was broken down by age of the respondent (Figure 5.1). There was a statistically significant age trend for both men and women, with more younger respondents having had their first sexual intercourse under the age of 16 years. Whereas 14% of male respondents in the 45–54 years age

Table 5.1. Percentage distribution of age (in years) at first intercourse by gender[1]

	Men (%)	Women (%)[2]
Under 16	25	14
16	18	18 *
17	15	18 *
18	12	16
19–21	17	23
22 and over	10	9 *
Not happened yet	3	3 *
Base:[3]	1 695	1 702

[1]SQ11 How old were you when you first had sexual intercourse with a man/woman?
[2]Chi-squared test for differences between men and women statistically significant p < 0.05 unless marked *
[3]Base: missing 9% men and 8% women

group had had sex before 16 years of age, 40% of 16- to 19-year-old men had done so. The trend for women was as striking (16- to 19-year-olds 29%; 45- to 54-year-olds 4%). The opposite age trend was apparent for those respondents who had their first sexual intercourse at the age of 19 years or above.

Age at first sexual intercourse was broken down by the respondent's occupational group (Figure 5.2). Men and women employed in manual occupations were more likely to have had their first sexual intercourse at an earlier age than respondents from non-manual occupations. The contrast was greatest for men: 30% of men in manual occupations had their first sexual intercourse under 16 years of age compared with 17% of those employed in non-manual occupations.

When age at first intercourse was broken down by the demographic cluster variable, those in the worse-off cluster (A) were statistically significantly more likely to have had their first sexual intercourse at an earlier age. Twenty-eight per cent of respondents in cluster A compared with 16% in cluster B had their first sexual intercourse under 16 years of age. Conversely 22% of cluster B had their first sexual intercourse at 19 to 21 years of age compared with 14% in cluster A.

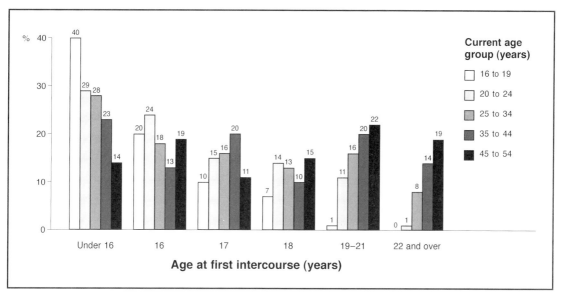

Mantel–Haenszel test for trend with age of respondent p < 0.05 for under 16, 19–21, 22 and over

(i) Men

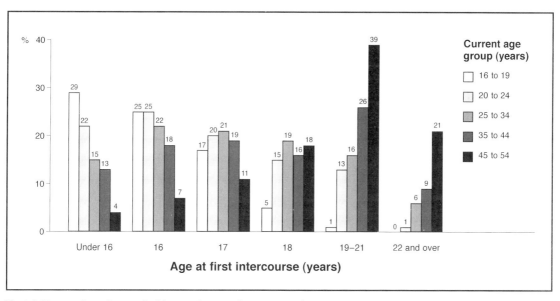

Mantel–Haenszel test for trend with age of respondent p < 0.05 for all

(ii) Women

Fig. 5.1. Percentage distribution of age at first sexual intercourse by gender by age of respondent

117

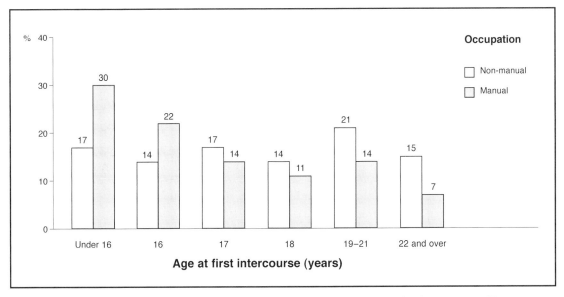

Chi-squared test for differences between occupational groups p < 0.05 except age at first intercourse – 17 years

(i) Men

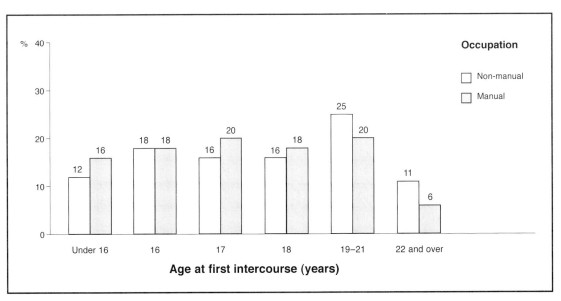

Chi-squared test for differences between occupational groups p < 0.05 for under 16, 19–21, 22 and over

(ii) Women

Fig. 5.2. Percentage distribution of age at first sexual intercourse by gender by occupational group

Sexual partners in the previous year

All respondents were asked the number of sexual partners they had had in the previous year (Table 5.2). The larger majority of men and women had had only one sexual partner in the previous year (72% of men, 82% of women). Men were more likely to have had more than one partner than women.

Table 5.2. Percentage distribution of the number of sexual partners in the previous year by gender[1]

	Men (%)	Women (%)[2]
None	10	9*
1	72	82
2	7	5
3	3	2
4	2	1
5	1	<1
6–10	2	<1
>10	2	1
Base:[3]	1 613	1 641

[1]SQ22 In the last 12 months, with how many women/men have you had vaginal sexual intercourse? Please include every woman/man you have had vaginal sexual intercourse with in the last 12 months, even if only once. Please remember to include your present partner (if you have had vaginal sexual intercourse with her/him). If you can't remember exactly please give your best estimate

[2]Chi-squared for differences between men and women statistically significant $p < 0.05$ unless marked *

[3]Base: those who have had sexual intercourse. Missing 11% men and 9% women

The number of sexual partners was broken down by age group for men and women separately (Figure 5.3(i)/(ii)). There was a statistically significant age trend for the proportion of respondents having more than two sexual partners. Whereas 55% of men aged 16 to 19 years had had sexual intercourse in the previous year with two or more partners, only 7% of men aged 45 to 54 years had done so.

The proportion of respondents who had had sexual intercourse with two or more partners in the previous year was higher in demographic cluster group A than group B (20% compared with 12%) (Figure 5.4).

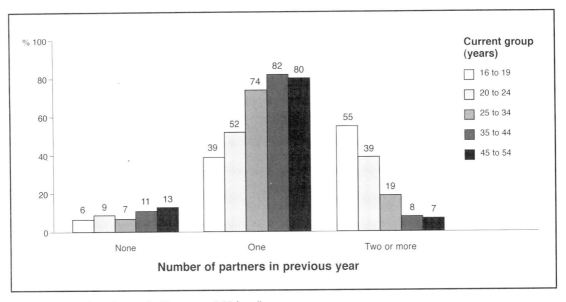

Mantel–Haenszel test for trend with age p < 0.05 for all

(i) Men

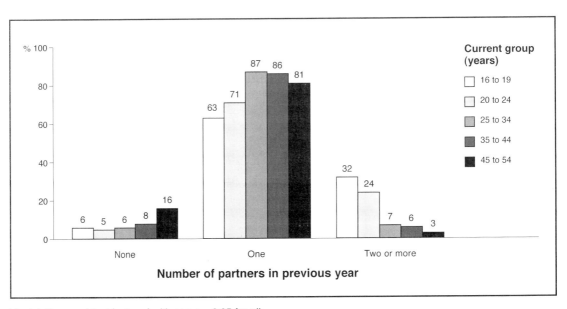

Mantel–Haenszel test for trend with age p < 0.05 for all

(ii) Women

Fig. 5.3. Percentage distribution of number of partners in the previous year by gender by age

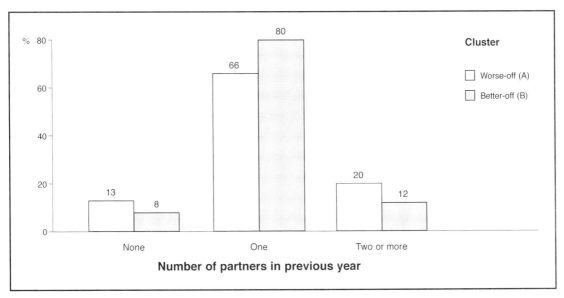

Chi-squared test for differences between cluster group p < 0.05 for all

Fig. 5.4. Percentage distribution of number of partners in the previous year by demographic cluster group

Men and women who had no sexual partners in the previous year were more likely to have had their first sexual intercourse at an older age than respondents who had had one or more partners in the previous year (Figure 5.5 (i)/(ii)). There were statistically significant trends with age at first intercourse for each level of number of partners (except for one partner in women).

Respondents were asked when they last had sexual intercourse, what kind of relationship they were in with that person (Table 5.3). Fifty-seven per cent of men and 64% of women were married to the person with whom they last had sex. A further 29% of men and 32% of women reported that they were either living with their partner or in a steady relationship. Men were more likely to have had sex with someone defined as not a steady partner at the time (men 12%; women 4%).

The number of partners respondents reported that they had in the previous year was broken down by the relationship the respondent had with the last person with whom they had had sexual intercourse (Figure 5.6(i)/(ii)). Men and women who were not in steady partnerships were more likely to have had two or more sexual partners in the last year (men – not steady and no partners 22%, not steady and two or more partners 58%; women – 12% and 52% respectively). Few married men and women reported having more than one sexual partner in the previous year; men and women in steady relationships, but not married were more likely to have had two or more partners in the previous year compared with those who were married or living together.

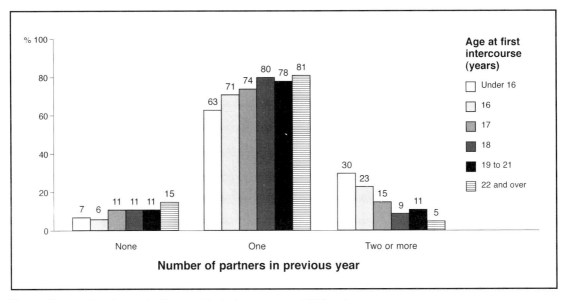

Mantel–Haenszel test for trend with age at first intercourse p < 0.05 for all

(i) Men

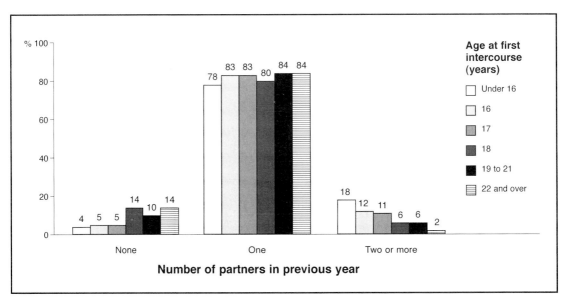

Mantel–Haenszel test for trend with age at first intercourse p < 0.05 for no and two or more partners

(ii) Women

Fig. 5.5. Percentage distribution of age at first sexual intercourse by gender by number of sexual partners in the previous year

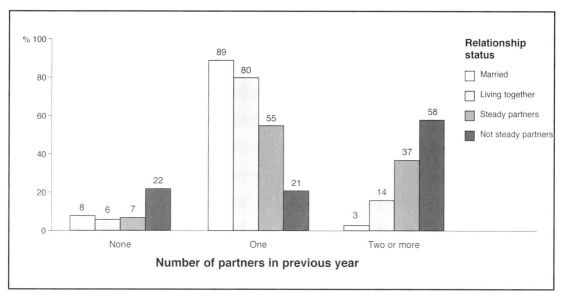

Mantel–Haenszel test for trend with relationship to last partner p < 0.05 for all

(i) Men

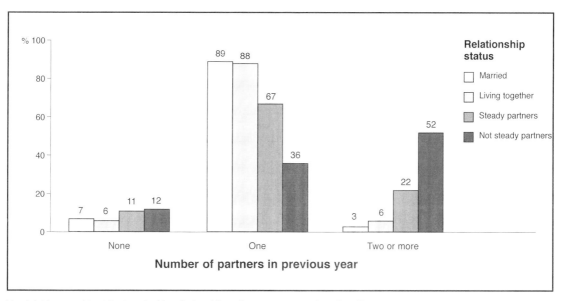

Mantel–Haenszel test for trend with relationship to last partner p < 0.05 for all

(ii) Women

Figure 5.6. Percentage distribution of number of partners in the previous year by gender by relationship to last partner

Table 5.3. Percentage distribution of the respondents' relationship with last sexual partner by gender[1]

	Men (%)	Women (%)[2]
Married together	57	64
Living together (not married)	9	12
Steady partners (not living together)	20	20 *
Not steady partners at the time	12	4
Can't remember	2	<1
Base:[3]	1 662	1 685

[1]SQ16 When you last had sexual intercourse, what kind of relationship were you in with this woman/man?
[2]Chi-squared test for differences between men and women statistically significant p < 0.05 unless marked *
[3]Base: those who have had sexual intercourse. Missing 8% men and 6% women

Knowledge and attitudes

This section explores the respondents' attitudes to sex education for children, and their perception of the adequacy of their own knowledge and information about sexual health issues.

- Two-thirds of men and women think sex education should be provided mainly by parents.
- The majority of men and women think that parents should be included by schools in sex education, women more so than men.
- Two-thirds of men and women do *not* think that TV adverts for AIDS and condoms should be restricted to after 9 pm.
- The inclusion of factual topics about sex and contraception in sex education is supported by most men and women. Women would like to see more inclusion of topics about feelings, emotions and personal choice.
- One-quarter of men and women thought homosexuality and lesbianism are very important to include in sex education lessons.
- Most men and women do not feel that they have adequate knowledge of emergency conception, recognising the symptoms of sexually transmitted diseases, or having an HIV test.

Attitudes to the provision of sex education

Respondents were asked whether they agreed with a series of statements about sex education (Table 5.4). Sixty-three per cent of men and 66% of women tended to agree or strongly agree that sex education should be provided mainly by parents. Eighty-three per cent of women and 75% of men (gender differences were statistically significant) either agreed or strongly agreed that parents should be included by schools in helping with sex education for their children. Nearly two-thirds of men and women disagreed with the statement that adverts for AIDS and condoms should not be shown on television before 9 pm. Men were more likely than women to think that schools were more important than parents when it came to sex education for young people (men agree or strongly agree – 43%; women – 33%).

Table 5.4. Percentage distribution of responses to statements about sex education by gender[1]

	(%) Strongly agree		(%) Tend to agree		(%) Tend to disagree		(%) Strongly disagree		(%) Don't know	
	M	W[2]	M	W	M	W	M	W	M	W
Sex education for young people should be provided mainly by parents[3]	20	23 †	43	43	26	26	8	6	4	2 †
Schools are more important than parents when it comes to sex education for young people[3]	14	10 †	29	23 †	43	50 †	12	14	3	3
Parents should be included by schools in helping with sex education for their children[3]	25	33 †	50	50	16	12 †	5	2 †	5	4
Adverts about AIDS and condoms should not be shown on television before 9 pm[3]	16	15	16	21 †	25	34 †	41	29 †	2	2
Most parents don't talk openly to their children about sexual matters[3]	31	27 †	55	57	8	9	2	3	4	5

[1]SQ1 Below are some statements about sex education. Please say how strongly you agree or disagree with each one.
[2]Chi-squared for differences between men and women statistically significant $p < 0.05$ if marked †
[3]Percentage missing 5 to 6% men and 3 to 6% women

As the age of respondents increased they were more likely to agree that sex education should be provided by parents (Figure 5.7). Men and women aged between 45 and 54 years of age, compared with those aged 16 to 19 years of age, were more likely to agree with the statement that sex education should be mainly provided by parents (men – 16–19 years 53%, 45–54 years 76%; women – 16–19 years 51%, 45–54 years 77%).

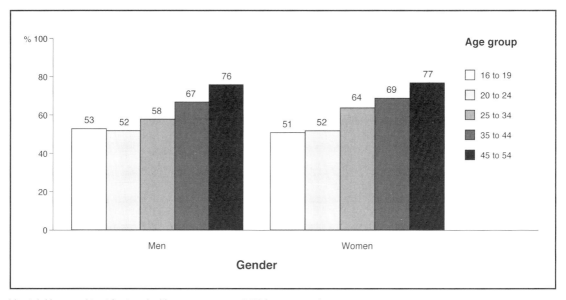

Mantel–Haenszel test for trend with age group p < 0.05 for men and women

Fig. 5.7. Percentage of respondents who agreed that 'Sex education should be provided mainly by parents' by gender by age group

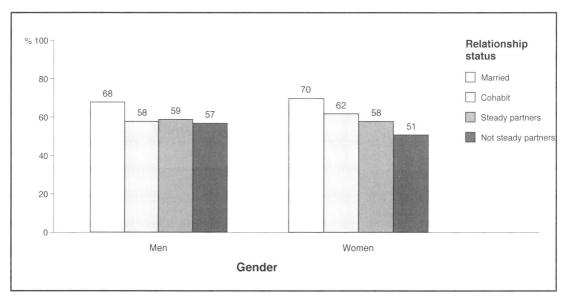

Chi-squared test for differences by relationship status p < 0.05 for married versus all other relationships

Fig. 5.8. Percentage of respondents who agreed that 'Sex education should be provided mainly by parents' by gender by relationship to last sexual partner

Figure 5.8 presents the proportion of respondents in agreement with the statement that sex education should be provided mainly by parents, broken down by the relationship of the respondent to their last partner. Married men and women were more likely to agree that sex education should be provided by parents than those respondents who were not in a steady relationship (married and 'not steady' men, 68% and 57% respectively; married and 'not steady' women, 70% and 51% – differences statistically significant).

As the age of respondents increased they were more likely to agree with the statement that parents should be included by schools in sex education. (Men – 16–19 62%, 45–54 83 %; women – 16–19 72%, 45–54 83% – age trends were statistically significant) (Figure 5.9).

The majority of respondents disagreed with the statement that adverts about AIDS should not be shown before 9 pm, but the proportion agreeing rose with increasing age of the respondent (men – 16–19 28%, 45–54 38%; women – 16–19 30%, 45–54 45%; age trends were significant) (Figure 5.10).

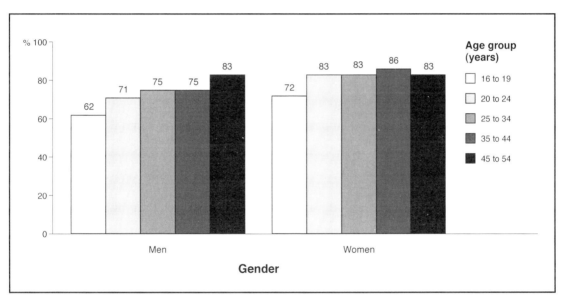

Mantel–Haenszel test for trend with age group p < 0.05 for men and women

Fig. 5.9. Percentage of respondents who agreed that 'Parents should be included by schools in sex education' by gender by age group

There were no statistically significant differences by the demographic cluster variable for agreement with statements about sex education, except for 'schools are more important than parents', where 42% of cluster A agreed in comparison to 37% of cluster B.

When respondents were asked how important they thought it was to include items from a list of topics in sex education in schools (Table 5.5), the majority

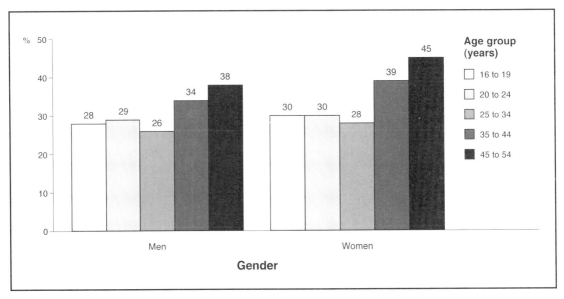

Mantel–Haenszel test for trend with age group p < 0.05 for men and women

Fig. 5.10. Percentage of respondents who agreed that 'Adverts about AIDS should not be shown before 9pm' by gender by age group

of both men and women thought the following topics were very important to include: human sexual reproduction (men 75%, women 81%); contraception and family planning (men 81%, women 87%); how to use a condom (men 66%, women 70%); how HIV (the AIDS virus) is passed on (men 86%, women 88%); how other STDs are passed on (men 82%, women 84%); how to talk to sexual partners about safer sex (men 59%, women 70%); women stated that these topics were very important, significantly more than men throughout (Table 5.5). Significantly more women also thought that how to express feelings and emotions in sexual relationships and how to make personal choices about having sexual relationships were very important (men 42% and 50% respectively; women 49% and 65% respectively). The majority of respondents considered it very important or fairly important to include homosexuality and lesbianism (men – very 24%, fairly 40%; women – very 28%, fairly 46%). Eighteen per cent of men and 14% of women considered it fairly important not to include these topics, and 10% and 5% respectively thought it very important not to include these subjects. All gender differences were statistically significant.

As shown in the previous section, age at first intercourse is decreasing, particularly for those in manual occupations, and contraceptive use is less likely at first intercourse for those in the 'worse-off' demographic cluster. This emphasises the need to continue to educate children under 16 about safer sex messages, through schools or the media. That this is likely to be acceptable is supported by the finding that the majority of respondents

Table 5.5. Percentage distribution of responses to statements about sex education in schools by gender[1]

	(%) Very important to include		(%) Fairly important to include		(%) Fairly important not to include		(%) Very important not to include		(%) Don't know	
	M	W[2]	M	W	M	W	M	W	M	W
Human sexual reproduction[3]	75	81 †	22	16 †	1	1	1	<1	2	1
Contraception and family planning[3]	81	87 †	17	12 †	1	1	<1	<1	1	<1
How to use a condom[3]	66	70 †	27	23 †	4	4	1	1	2	2
Homosexuality and lesbianism[3]	24	28 †	40	46 †	18	14 †	10	5 †	8	7
How HIV (the AIDS virus) is passed on[3]	86	88 †	12	11	1	<1	1	<1	<1	<1 †
How other sexually transmitted diseases are passed on[3]	82	84 †	16	14	1	1	1	1	1	1
How to express feelings and emotions in sexual relationships[3]	42	49 †	38	38	11	7 †	3	2 †	5	4
How to talk to sexual partners about safer sex[3]	59	70 †	31	25 †	5	3 †	2	1 †	2	1 †
How to make personal choices about having sexual relationships[3]	50	65 †	33	27 †	9	4 †	3	2 †	5	3 †

[1]SQ2 For each of the following topics, please say how important you think it is that each one should or should not be included in sex education in schools
[2]Chi-squared test for differences between men and women statistically significant $p < 0.05$ if marked †
[3]Missing 2 to 5% men and 2 to 4% women

agreed that contraception should be included in school sex education. Increased parental involvement is clearly supported by these findings. Further indication of the increased social acceptability of education on these issues is given by the findings that the majority of respondents thought that television adverts about AIDS and condoms should be screened before the 9 pm watershed.

Personal knowledge and information

Significantly more women than men felt they had adequate knowledge of information about contraception and birth control (men 93%, women 96%); emergency contraception (men 26%, women 42%); how to express your love/feelings to your partner (men 74%, women 78%), how to express better to your partner your sexual needs (men 55%, women 59%) and how to raise the subject of safer sex (men 64%, women 68%). Only about a third of respondents felt they had adequate knowledge or information about

Table 5.6. Percentage distribution of respondents' knowledge or information about sexual health issues by gender[1]

	Men (%)	Women(%)[2]
Contraception/birth control	93	96 †
Emergency ('morning after') contraception	26	42 †
Ways in which HIV (the AIDS virus) can be passed on	85	85
Ways in which other sexually transmitted diseases can be passed on	74	75
Recognising symptoms of sexually transmitted disease	31	33
Having a blood test for the AIDS virus (HIV test)	47	46
How to express your love/feelings to your partner	74	78 †
How to express better to a partner your sexual needs	55	59 †
How to satisfy the sexual needs of your partner	69	67
How to raise the subject of safer sex	64	68 †
None of these	2	1
Base:[3]	1 813	1 822

[1]SQ3 Which of these items do you think you have adequate knowledge or information about? Multiple response question
[2]Chi-squared test for differences between men and women statistically significant $p < 0.05$ if marked †
[3]Base: missing 3% men and 1% women

emergency contraception and recognising the symptoms of sexually transmitted diseases, and less than one-half about having a blood test for the AIDS virus (Table 5.6).

When relationship status was taken into account there were significant differences in the proportion of men that felt adequately informed: between married and cohabiting men for emergency contraception (22% and 37%), between married versus men in a steady relationship for emergency contraception (22% and 36%), HIV transmission (84% and 89%) and STD transmission (77% and 71%); between cohabiting men versus those in a steady relationship for STD transmission (80% and 71%) and symptoms of STD (40% and 29%); between cohabiting men versus those not in a steady relationship for emergency contraception (37% and 26%); and between men in steady and not steady relationships for emergency contraception (36% and 26%), how to express sexual needs (60% and 51%) and how to raise the subject of safer sex (71% and 60%).

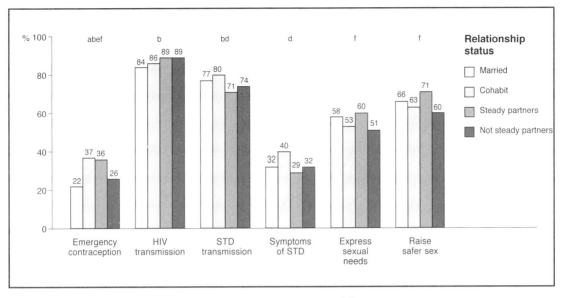

Chi-squared test for differences between relationship status p < 0.05 as follows:
[a]married v. cohabit; [b]married v. steady; [c]married v. not steady; [d]cohabit v. steady; [e]cohabit v. not steady; [f]steady v. not steady

(i) Men

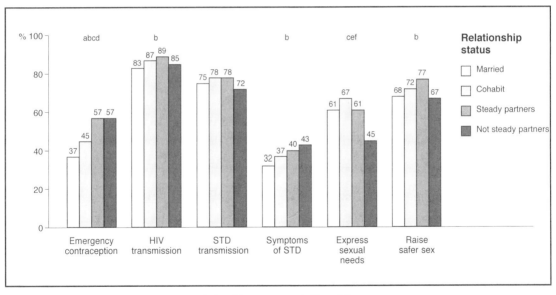

Chi-squared test for differences between relationship status p < 0.05 as follows:
[a]married v. cohabit; [b]married v. steady; [c]married v. not steady; [d]cohabit v. steady; [e]cohabit v. not steady; [f]steady v. not steady

(ii) Women

Fig. 5.11. Percentage of respondents feeling adequately informed about each sexual health issue by gender by relationship status

Figure 5.11(i)/(ii) demonstrates similar significant differences between relationship status regarding the proportions of female respondents who felt adequately informed about these topics. Significantly fewer married women than those in a steady relationship felt adequately informed about emergency contraception (37% and 57%), HIV transmission (83% and 89%), symptoms of STD (32% and 40%), and how to raise the subject of safer sex (68% and 77%). Fewer married women than those cohabiting and those not in a steady relationship felt adequately informed about emergency contraception (married 37%; cohabiting 45%; not steady 57%). More married women than those not in a steady relationship felt informed about how to express sexual needs (61% and 45%). Significantly fewer women cohabiting were informed about emergency contraception than those in either a steady, or not steady relationship (cohabiting 45%, steady 57%; not steady 57%). Cohabiting women and those in a steady relationship were more likely to feel adequately informed about how to express their sexual needs than women not in a steady relationship (cohabiting 67%, steady 61%; not steady 45% respectively).

The proportion of respondents feeling adequately informed about sexual health issues was broken down by HIV risk score for men and women (Figure 5.12(i)/(ii)) (see 'Condom use in relation to HIV risk' below for details of how this risk score was computed). There were not statistically significant differences in subjects' responses, although trends were seen towards male respondents at higher risk being more likely to feel they had adequate knowledge of HIV transmission than those respondents at lower risk (high 89%, moderate 94%, low 85%); the opposite trend was apparent for women (high 78%, moderate 88%, low 86%).

When the proportion feeling that they had adequate knowledge about emergency contraception was broken down by age (Figure 5.13) there was a statistically significant trend to decreasing perceptions of adequacy of knowledge with increasing age (16–19, men 38% and women 61%; 45–54, men 16% and women 31%). There was no trend for adequacy of knowledge about expressing personal sexual needs with age for men or women (Figure 5.14).

Respondents in demographic cluster A (worse-off) versus cluster B (better-off), felt less adequately informed on all subjects except emergency contraception. Statistically significant differences were seen between clusters A and B for contraception/birth control (90% and 95% respectively); transmission of HIV (83% and 86%), transmission of STDs (72% and 75%), how to express love/feelings (68% and 79%), how to express sexual needs (51% and 58%), and how to satisfy sexual needs (60% and 71%).

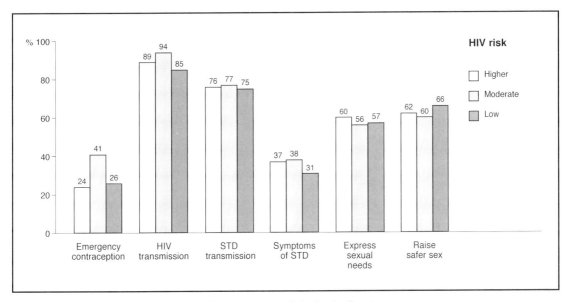

Mantel–Haenszel test for trend with HIV risk group none statistically significant

(i) Men

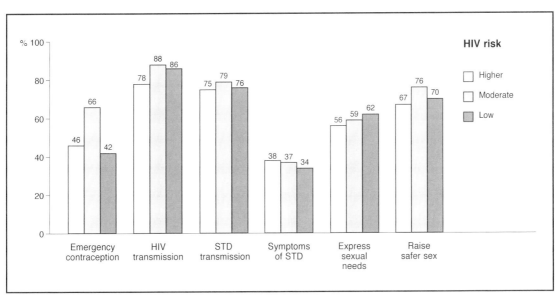

Mantel–Haenszel test for trend with HIV risk group none statistically significant

(ii) Women

Fig. 5.12. Percentage of respondents feeling adequately informed about each sexual health issue by gender by HIV risk

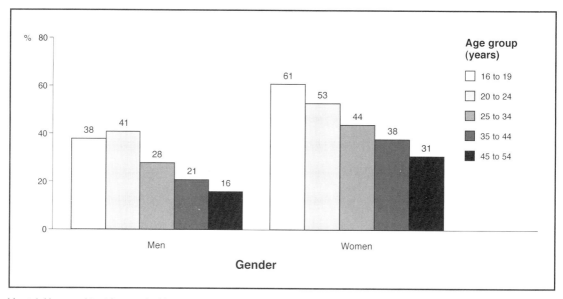

Mantel–Haenszel test for trend with age group p < 0.05 for men and women

Fig. 5.13. Percentage of respondents feeling adequately informed about emergency contraception by gender by age group

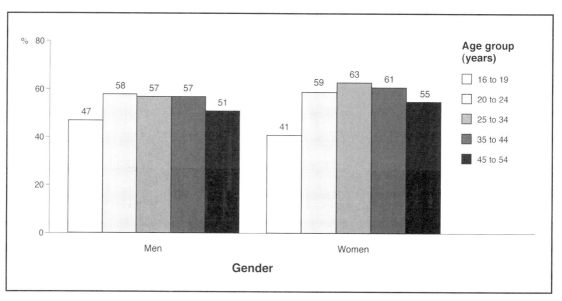

Mantel–Haenszel test for trend with age group, none statistically significant

Fig. 5.14. Percentage of respondents feeling adequately informed about expressing their personal sexual needs by gender by age group

Contraception and condom use

This section explores contraceptive use at first and last sexual intercourse, and reasons for not using condoms. A risk score for HIV is computed from the number of sexual partners and the frequency of use of condoms, and barriers to condom use are assessed against estimated HIV risk.

- More women (19%) than men (16%) report not using any contraceptives the last time that they had sex.

- A fifth of men and women did not use any contraceptives the first time that they had sex. For those whose first intercourse was more recent (1991–93) this has reduced to 5–6%.

- Barrier methods of contraception are more often used at first intercourse than other methods, and their use is increasing. Around three-quarters of men and women in 1991–93 report using condoms at first intercourse.

- People who are 'worse off' are less likely to use contraception at first intercourse than those who are 'better off'.

- People in steady relationships tend to stop using condoms, and increasingly use the pill over time.

- Men not in steady relationships continue to use condoms, but women tend not to and change to the pill.

- Men and women are most likely not to use condoms because they 'forget to carry them' or 'get carried away in the heat of the moment'.

- People not in steady relationships thought they were more likely not to use condoms because they forget to carry them.

- A computed HIV risk score indicated that 5% of men and 3% of women are at high risk of contracting HIV; younger and manual workers and those in the 'worse-off' cluster were at higher risk.

- Of those who had two or more partners in the last year, women and older respondents are at higher risk.

- Men and women at higher risk of HIV were more likely to forget to carry condoms, and to get carried away in the heat of the moment.

- All factors stopping condom use, including cost, were higher for the 'worse-off' group.

- Potentially neglected by safer sex campaigns are a higher-risk group of older men having 'affairs'.

Table 5.7. Percentage distribution of respondents' method of contraception used when last had sexual intercourse by gender[1]

	Men (%)	Women (%)[2]
The pill	28	29
Emergency ('morning after') contraception	<1	<1
The coil/IUD/intra-uterine device	4	5
The female condom	<1	<1
Condom/sheath/Durex	30	22 †
Cap/diaphragm/Dutch cap	1	1
Foam tablets/jellies/creams	<1	<1
Suppositories/pessaries/aerosol foam	<1	<1
Sponge	0	<1
Douching/washing	<1	<1
Safe period/rhythm method	1	1
Withdrawal	5	4
Sterilisation/vasectomy	19	23 †
Other method of protection	2	2
None	16	19 †
Can't remember	1	<1 †
Base:[3]	1 655	1 673

[1] SQ17 When you last had sexual intercourse with a woman/man, which of these if any were used? Multiple response question
[2] Chi-squared test for differences between men and women statistically significant p < 0.05 if marked †
[3] Base: those who have had sexual intercourse missing 8% men and 7% women

Contraception at last and first intercourse

All those respondents who had ever had sexual intercourse with a woman/man were asked which, if any, of a list of contraceptive methods were employed on the last occasion that they had had sexual intercourse (Table 5.7). About a third of respondents used the pill (men 28%, women 29%); 30% of men and 22% of women used a condom (gender difference statistically significant), and 19% of men and 23% of women used sterilisation or vasectomy (gender difference statistically significant). Statistically significantly more women (19%) than men (16%) reported not having used any form of contraception. The proportion of men and women who reported using no contraception at last intercourse was consistent with that reported by Wellings *et al.* (1994) in relation to methods of contraception used in the past year.

The pattern of contraceptive usage differed from that seen when respondents were asked about the form of contraception used, if any, on the first time that they had sexual intercourse (Table 5.8). Fewer men and women used the pill

Table 5.8. Percentage distribution of method of contraception, if used, at first sexual intercourse by gender[1]

	Men (%)	Women (%)[2]
The pill	22	21
The female condom	1	1
Condom/sheath/Durex	37	46 †
Other contraception	3	1 †
He/I withdrew	10	11
Made sure it was a 'safe period'	3	2 †
No precautions by me, don't know about partner	6	<1 †
No precautions by either of us	22	20
Can't remember	5	4
Don't know	2	1 †
Base:[3]	1 661	1 677

[1]SQ12 Did you or your partner use any form of contraception or take any precautions that first time, or not? Multiple response question
[2]Chi-squared test for difference between men and women statistically significant p < 0.05 if marked †
[3]Base: those who have had sexual intercourse. Missing 8% men and 7% women

(22% and 21% respectively) and more relied on the condom at first intercourse (37% men and 46% women – gender difference statistically significant). Whereas on the last occasion only 5% of men and 4% of women reported withdrawal as a method of contraception, on the first occasion 10% of men and 11% of women relied on this method. Use of no precautions was also higher, 6% of men used no precautions themselves and did not know whether their partner did, for women this was <1% (gender differences statistically significant). However, about a fifth of both men and women admitted that neither they nor their partner used any precautions on the first occasion they had intercourse (men 22%, women 20%).

The public health significance of these results needs to be considered in the context of whether respondents are likely to be at higher risk of HIV. A risk score has been calculated; this is a composite of the number of sexual partners (Table 5.2) and frequency of use of condoms (presented later as Table 5.10). Subjects were defined as high risk if they had multiple partners and had not used a condom in the last year (Table 5.9). Men were more likely than women to be at high risk (5% compared with 3%) and overall about 10% of men and 6% of women were at either moderate or high risk.

Table 5.9. Percentage distribution of respondents' computed risk of HIV by gender[1]

	Men (%)	Women (%)[2]
Higher	5	3 *
Moderate	5	3
Low	91	94
Base:[3]	1 616	1 647

[1]Computed HIV risk from SQ22 and SQ26
[2]Chi-squared test for differences between men and women statistically significant p < 0.05 unless marked *
[3]Base: those who have had sexual intercourse. Missing 11% men and 8% women

Respondents' computed risk of HIV was broken down by broad age (Figure 5.15). Younger respondents were more likely to be at moderate risk of HIV than older respondents (11% compared with 2% statistically significant). There was no statistically significant regional variation in the relationship reported above.

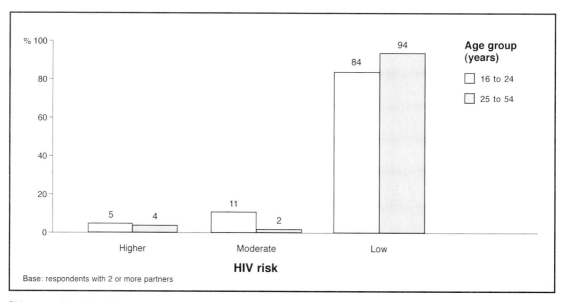

Chi-squared test for differences between age groups p < 0.05 for moderate and low risk

Fig. 5.15. Percentage distribution of computed risk of HIV by age of respondent

Respondents who were not living together were more likely to be at higher risk of HIV than those who were living together with their partner (Figure 5.16). This difference was apparent for both higher (8% compared with 2%) and moderate (11% compared with 1%) risk.

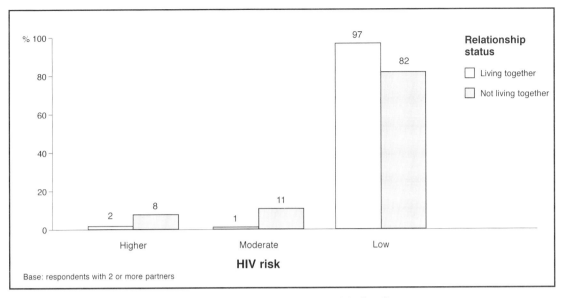

Base: respondents with 2 or more partners

Chi-squared test for differences between relationship status groups p < 0.05 for all

Fig. 5.16. Percentage distribution of computed risk of HIV by relationship status

The relationship between age at first sexual intercourse and the method of contraception for men and women is explored in Figure 5.17(i)/(ii). Use of a barrier method of contraception at first sexual intercourse was reported more commonly than any other method by men and women, regardless of the age at which they had had first intercourse (no statistically significant age trends). (Barrier methods included female condom and cap/diaphragm but were mostly condoms.) Use of the pill at first intercourse significantly increased among men and women as age at first intercourse increased (men <16 – 14%, 22+ – 33%; women <16 – 14%, 22+ – 29%). There was a statistically significant decrease in the proportion of both men and women reporting using no contraception as age at first intercourse increased (men <16 – 33%, 22+ – 16%; women <16 – 30%, 22+ – 22%).

From the respondents' replies regarding their age at first intercourse, the data were re-analysed using the year during which first intercourse took place as a variable to see if there was any trend in the use of contraception over time (Figure 5.18(i)/(ii)). It should be noted that older respondents were being asked to think back over 30–40 years. The use of barrier methods of contraception at first sexual intercourse has increased consistently amongst men and women since 1981. While only 34% of men and 49% of women whose first sexual intercourse took place between 1981 and 1985 used a barrier method, these proportions had significantly increased to 72% and 79% respectively by 1991–93. The proportion of respondents reporting that they did not use any method of contraception at first sexual intercourse significantly declined during this period (1981–85: men 21%, women 14%; 1991–93: men 5%, women 6%). Use of the pill has remained relatively constant during this period.

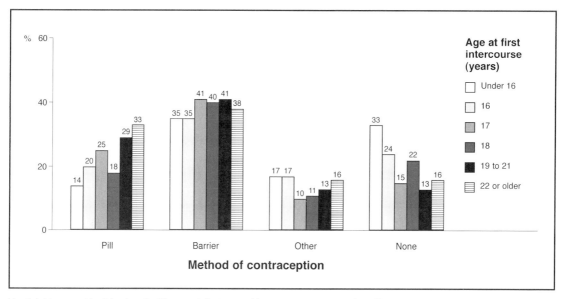

Mantel–Haenszel test for trend with age at first sexual intercourse p < 0.05 for pill and none

(i) Men

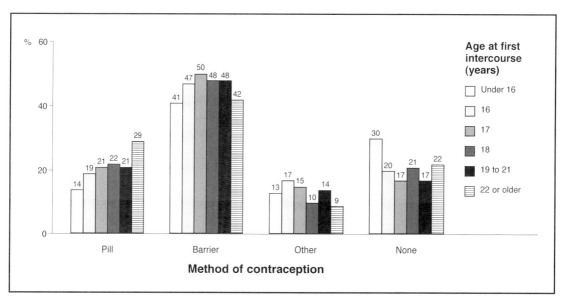

Mantel–Haenszel test for trend with age at first sexual intercourse p < 0.05 for pill and none

(ii) Women

Fig. 5.17. Percentage distribution of age at first sexual intercourse by method of contraception at first sexual intercourse by gender

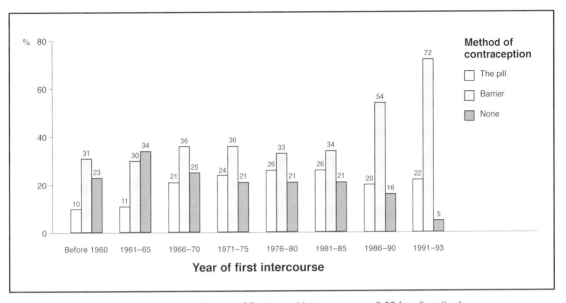

Manel–Haenszel test for trend with calendar year of first sexual intercourse p < 0.05 for all methods

(i) Men

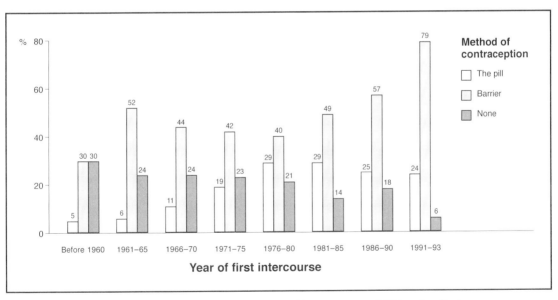

Mantel–Haenszel test for trend with calendar year of first sexual intercourse p < 0.05 for all methods

(ii) Women

Fig. 5.18. Percentage distribution of calendar year of first intercourse by method of contraception at first intercourse by gender

While the above demonstrated an increase in the use of condoms at first sexual intercourse since 1981, it may be that this behaviour was not sustained with subsequent partners. The responses to use of condoms at first and most recent intercourse were collated for those with either a steady or not steady current partner for men and women (Figure 5.19(i)/(ii)). For men in a current steady relationship there was a non-statistically significant decline in use of condoms at the first time and at the last time from 53% to 49%, and a larger increase in use of the pill, from 19% to 51%. Conversely, condom usage at first and last intercourse has increased amongst men not in a steady relationship from 46% to 62%, and also the use of the pill has increased from first to last time in this group, from 15% to 30% (all differences were statistically significant).

For women in steady relationships there has been a sharper decline in condom use, at both first and last sexual intercourse from 66% to 39%, and a greater increase in use of the pill (21% and 64%). For women who were not in a steady relationship the pattern for first and last intercourse was similar, with no reduction in condom use and a statistically significant increase in use of the pill (52% and 51%; 26% and 44% respectively).

This decline in use of barrier methods with sexual experience has been shown for both men and women in steady relationships. The increase in condom use for men not in steady relationships is in line with safer sex messages. Use for women has remained constant at 52% and 51%, and demonstrates the need to continue to emphasise the multiple benefits of barrier methods in relation to STDs as well as contraception.

When contraceptive method at first sexual intercourse was examined by the demographic cluster variable, it was clear that cluster group A (the younger, lower income, less-educated group) used the pill at first intercourse significantly more than cluster group B (better-off and more educated) (25% compared with 20%) and condoms significantly less than cluster group B (38% and 43%). Cluster group A were less likely than cluster group B to use contraceptives at first intercourse (25% and 20%) (Figure 5.20).

Table 5.10 presents the distribution of use of condoms in the last 12 months when having intercourse. Over half of all respondents (55% men, 63% women) never used condoms in the last year; 27% of men and 22% of women always or most times used a condom.

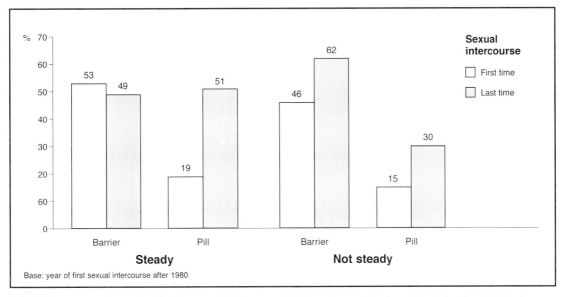

Paired Wilcoxon test for method first time and last time p < 0.05 for all except barrier methods for those in steady relationships

(i) Men

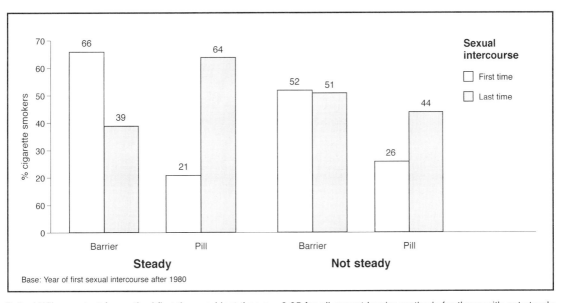

Paired Wilcoxon test for method first time and last time p < 0.05 for all except barrier methods for those with not steady relationships

(ii) Women

Fig. 5.19. Percentage distribution of condom use at first and most recent sexual intercourse by relationship to last partner by gender

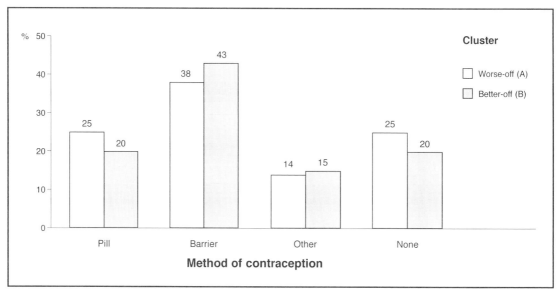

Chi-squared test for differences between cluster groups p < 0.05 except for 'other'

Fig. 5.20. Percentage distribution of method of contraception used at first sexual intercourse by demographic cluster group

Table 5.10. Percentage distribution of respondents' use of condoms when having intercourse in the past 12 months by gender[1]

	Men (%)	Women (%)[2]
Always	16	14 *
Most times	11	8
About half the time	5	3
Occasionally	13	12 *
Never	55	63
Base:[3]	1 527	1 523

[1] SQ26 Thinking of the occasions when you had sexual intercourse in the last 12 months, how often did you use condoms?
[2] Chi-squared test for differences between men and women statistically significant p < 0.05 unless marked *
[3] Base: those who have had sexual intercourse. Missing 15% men and 15% women

Reasons for not using condoms

Respondents who had ever had sexual intercourse were asked how likely each of a list of factors would stop them using condoms if they wished to use them (Table 5.10). For men and women the factors that emerged as fairly likely or very likely to stop them using condoms were: forgetting to carry

Table 5.11. Percentage distribution of respondents' statements which might stop people using condoms by gender[1]

	(%) Very unlikely		(%) Fairly unlikely		(%) Fairly likely		(%) Very likely	
	M	W[2]	M	W	M	W	M	W
Feeling embarrassed to buy condoms[3]	64	58 †	23	24	9	11	4	7 †
Forgetting to carry them[3]	30	35 †	31	34 †	29	22 †	11	9 †
Difficulty in using a condom[3]	63	50 †	26	34 †	8	11 †	4	5
The cost of condoms[3]	68	59 †	22	28 †	6	8 †	4	4
Difficulty in obtaining condoms[3]	67	62 †	25	29 †	5	6	3	3
Getting carried away in the heat of the moment[3]	28	28	32	33	30	27	11	12
Difficulty in talking about using condoms[3]	55	52	32	35	10	9	3	5
Your partner getting angry if you suggested using condoms[3]	56	61 †	33	28 †	7	7	4	4
Fears of giving a bad impression about your own sexual behaviour if you suggested using condoms[3]	53	62 †	33	29 †	6	6	3	4
Difficulty in planning ahead for sex[3]	46	47	35	33	14	14	5	7 †

[1]SQ42 How likely is it that each of the following would stop you using condoms, even if you wished to use them?
[2]Chi-squared test for differences between men and women statistically significant $p < 0.05$ if marked †
[3]Base: those who have had sexual intercourse. Missing 13 to16% men and 19 to 21% women

them (men 40%; women 31%); getting carried away in the heat of the moment (men 41%; women 39%); difficulty in planning ahead for sex (men 19%; women 21%) and difficulty in talking about using condoms (men 13%; women 14%). Significantly more women than men were very likely to be stopped from using condoms by feeling embarrassed to buy them (men 4%; women 7%) although the majority of men and women were very unlikely to be put off using condoms because they felt embarrassed buying them (men 64%, women 58%). Significantly more women were fairly likely to be stopped from using condoms because of difficulty in using them (men 8%; women 11%). Cost of condoms and difficulty in obtaining them did not seem to be major factors in determining whether they were used or not (very likely 4% and 3% respectively).

When forgetting to carry condoms as a cause for not using condoms was explored further by the type of relationship respondents were currently in, it was clear that significantly more men and women in non-steady relationships thought that forgetting to carry condoms was likely to prevent their use (48%

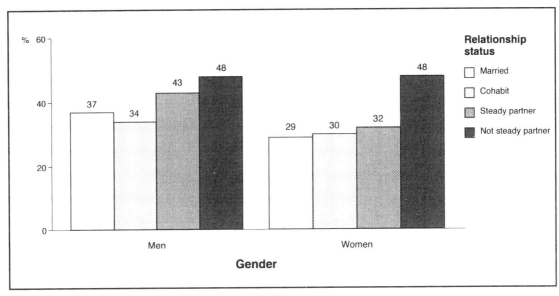

Mantel–Haenszel test for trend with relationship status p < 0.05 for men and women

Fig. 5.21. Percentage of respondents reporting 'Forgetting to carry condoms' as a likely cause of not using a condom by type of relationship by gender

for men and women, compared with steady partners 43% and 32% for women) (Figure 5.21). The trends for both men and women with relationship status were statistically significant. There was little difference in the response between those who were married and those who were living together.

Condom use in relation to HIV risk

The computed risk of HIV was also higher in respondents who were employed in manual occupations (Figure 5.22). The HIV risk score was also broken down by the demographic cluster (Figure 5.23). Respondents in cluster A were over twice as likely to be at higher risk than respondents in cluster B (7% compared with 3%).

Respondents who had two or more partners in the last year were investigated further by occupational groups, living status, age, gender and region (Table 5.12). Those respondents who were living with a partner, but had more than one sexual partner (even though there were relatively few such people) were at very much higher risk than those not living with their current partner (60% compared with 20%). Further, women and older respondents with more than one sexual partner were also more likely to be at higher risk (women 38%, men 25%; 25–54 years 44%, 16–24 years 14%). These results suggest that these small groups are at particular risk, and given the focus of much sexual health education, likely to be missed. Previous research has highlighted the higher risk of older divorced men (Wellings *et al.*, 1994).

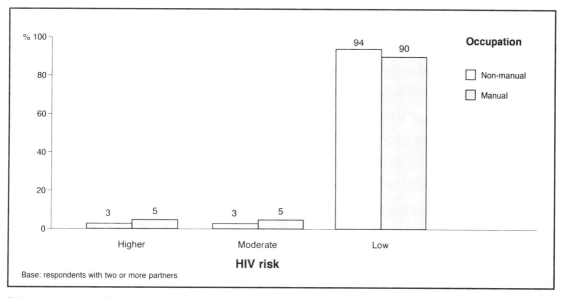

Chi-squared test for differences between occupational groups p < 0.05 for all

Fig. 5.22. Percentage distribution of computed risk of HIV by occupational group

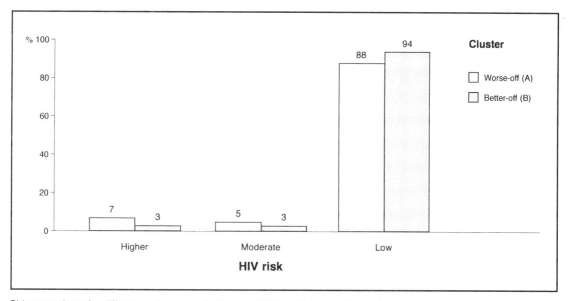

Chi-squared test for differences between clusters p < 0.05 for higher and low-risk groups

Fig. 5.23. Percentage distribution of computed risk of HIV by demographic cluster group

Table 5.12. Percentage distribution of HIV risk by occupation, relationship, age, gender and region – selected respondents with two or more partners

	HIV risk[1]		
	Higher (%)	Moderate (%)	Low (%)
Occupation			
Non-manual	30	26	44
Manual	32	32	36
Relationship			
Living together	60 †	23	17 †
Not living together	20	30	50
Age			
16–24 years	14 †	32	55 †
25–54 years	44	24	31
Gender			
Men	25 †	27	48 †
Women	38	30	33
Region			
North	25	26	50 †
Midlands	28	28	45
South	33	29	38

[1]Chi-squared test for differences between respondent categories within demographic variables and HIV risk category $p < 0.05$ if marked †

Selected factors were then explored by risk of HIV for men and women. For both men and women there was a significant relationship between increasing risk from HIV infection (as defined by HIV risk score) and increasing likelihood of forgetting to carry condoms (Figure 5.24). Both men and women (men 55%, women 62%) at higher risk were more likely to forget to carry condoms in comparison to those at low risk (men 37%, women 29%) (Figure 5.24). Those respondents who considered that difficulties in talking about condoms were likely to prevent their use were at higher risk of HIV (Figure 5.25). Twenty-five per cent of women and 23% of men at high risk were likely to have difficulties in talking about condom use compared with 13% and 12% respectively for respondents at low risk.

Difficulties in planning ahead were likely to prevent condom use particularly in women (46% of women) but also in men (29%) at higher risk of HIV, compared with women and men at low risk (19% and 17% respectively) (Figure 5.26).

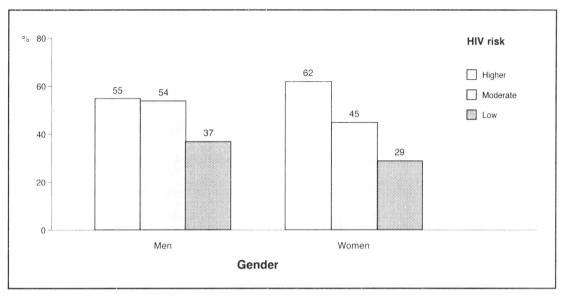

Mantel–Haenszel test for trend with HIV risk p < 0.05 for men and women

Fig. 5.24. Percentage of respondents who reported that 'Forgetting to carry condoms' was a likely cause of not using a condom by risk of HIV by gender

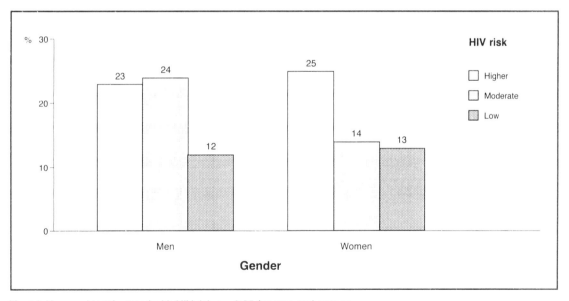

Mantel–Haenszel test for trend with HIV risk p < 0.05 for men and women

Fig. 5.25. Percentage of respondents who reported that 'Difficulties in talking about condom use' was a likely cause of not using a condom by risk of HIV by gender

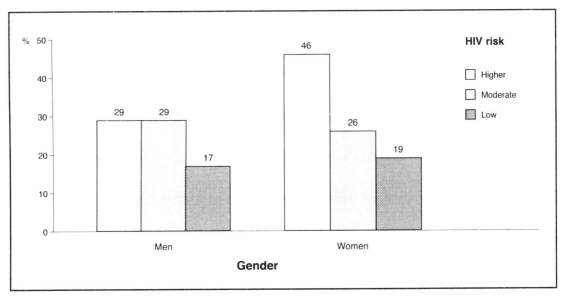

Mantel–Haenszel test for trend with HIV risk p < 0.05 for men and women

Fig. 5.26. Percentage of respondents who reported that 'Difficulties in planning ahead' was a likely cause of not using a condom by risk of HIV

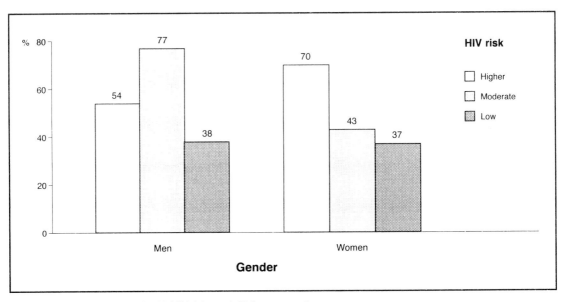

Mantel-Haenszel test for trend with HIV risk p < 0.05 for men and women

Fig. 5.27. Percentage of respondents reporting 'Getting carried away in the heat of the moment' as a likely cause of not using a condom by gender

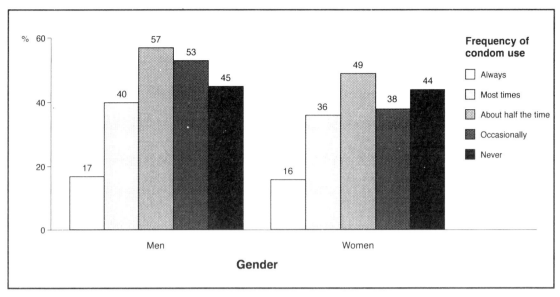

Mantel–Haenszel test for trend with frequency of condom use p < 0.05 for men and women

Fig. 5.28. Percentage of respondents reporting 'Getting carried away in the heat of the moment' as a likely cause of not using a condom by frequency of condom use by gender

There were also significant trends with HIV risk for those likely to stop using condoms because they got carried away in the heat of the moment (Figure 5.27). Seventy per cent of women and 54% of men at higher risk of HIV thought this was likely in comparison to 38% of men and 37% women at low risk. Respondents who reported using condoms either always or most times, were significantly more unlikely to state that getting carried away in the heat of the moment would stop them using them. In contrast, those using them half the time, occasionally or never, were more likely to get carried away in the heat of the moment (men – always 17%, half 57%, never 45%; women – always 16%, half 49%, never 44% (Figure 5.28).

Difficulties in using condoms were likely to prevent their use in 36% of higher-risk women and 26% of higher-risk men in comparison to 15% and 10% of low-risk women and men (trend statistically significant) (Figure 5.29).

The likelihood of factors stopping condom use were analysed by cluster groups (Table 5.13). There was a consistently significantly higher likelihood of all the factors stopping use of condoms for the worse-off cluster group in comparison with the 'better-educated, better-off' cluster group B. In cluster A cost was a factor for 20% of respondents compared with 9% in cluster B.

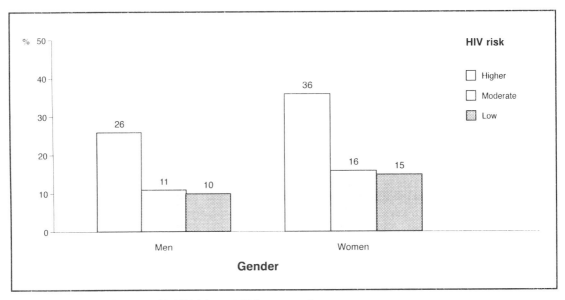

Mantel–Haenszel test for trend with HIV risk p < 0.05 for men and women

Fig. 5.29. Percentage of respondents reporting 'Difficulties in using condoms' was a likely cause of not using a condom by risk of HIV by gender

Table 5.13. Percentage of respondents stating factors likely to stop them using condoms by demographic cluster

	Cluster Worse-off (%)	Cluster Better-off (%)[1]
Feeling embarrassed to buy condoms	19	15
Forgetting to carry them with you	39	34
Difficulty in using a condom	18	13
The cost of condoms	20	9
Difficulty in obtaining condoms	13	8
Getting carried away in the heat of the moment	46	38
Difficulty in talking about using condoms	18	13
Your partner getting angry if you suggested using condoms	14	10
Fear of giving a bad impression about your own sexual behaviour if you suggested using a condom	13	8
Difficulty in planning ahead for sex	26	18

[1]Chi-squared test for differences between clusters p < 0.05 for all

Personal perceptions and risk of HIV

- About three-quarters of men and women felt they were not at all at risk of HIV or STDs.

- Men and women at higher and moderate risk of HIV underestimate their personal risk. Nearly one-half of those at higher risk think their sex life is not at all risky.

- About a quarter of men and a fifth of women are worried about getting HIV.

- More people in the 'worse-off' group are worried about getting HIV, and are in fact at higher risk.

- Very few people have sought voluntary testing for HIV and they do not differ by risk group.

All respondents were asked how much at risk they personally felt they were of becoming infected with HIV and other sexually transmitted diseases with their present sexual lifestyle (Table 5.14). The perception of risk was similar for HIV and STD. Seventy-one per cent of men and 79% of women felt not at all at risk of HIV, and 24% of men and 17% of women felt not very much at risk of infection with HIV (gender differences significant).

For other sexually transmitted diseases, 69% of men and 79% of women felt not at all at risk, and 25% of men and 17% of women felt not very much at risk (gender differences significant).

Table 5.14. Percentage distribution of perceived risk of HIV and sexually transmitted diseases by gender

	HIV[1]		STD[2]	
	Men (%)[3]	Women (%)[3]	Men (%)	Women (%)
Greatly at risk	1	1	1	<1
Quite a lot at risk	2	1	2	1†
Not very much at risk	24	17 †	25	17 †
Not at all at risk	71	79 †	69	79 †
Don't know	2	2	3	2
Base:	1 831[4]	1 797	1 831[5]	1 791

[1] SQ6 With your present sexual lifestyle, how much at risk do you personally feel of becoming infected with HIV (the AIDS virus)?
[2] SQ7 With your present sexual lifestyle, how much at risk do you personally feel of becoming infected with other sexually transmitted diseases?
[3] Chi-squared test for differences between men and women for HIV and STD separately statistically significant p < 0.05 if marked †
[4] Missing 2% men and 2% women
[5] Missing 2% men and 3% women

153

Table 5.15. Percentage distribution of blood tests for the AIDS virus (HIV test) by gender[1]

	Men (%)	Women (%)[2]
No	96	97
Base:[3]	1 621	1 617

[1]SQ29 Have you ever gone on your own initiative to have a blood test for the AIDS virus (HIV test)?
[2]Chi-squared test for differences between men and women not statistically significant
[3]Base: those who have had sexual intercourse. Missing 10% men and 10% women

Data for men and women were combined due to small numbers of respondents in the higher risk categories for HIV. When compared with their actual risk, men and women at higher and moderate risk underestimated their personal risk (Figure 5.30). Forty-nine per cent of those at higher risk perceived that their personal sexual lifestyle placed them at no risk at all, and a further 43% felt not very much at risk. Of those at moderate risk 28% perceived no personal risk at all, and 61% not very much risk. (Higher actual risk in comparison to low actual risk significant for each perceived risk level.)

When respondents were asked about their agreement with the statement that getting HIV was something that worried them about their sexual lifestyle these days, significantly more men than women agreed (26% and 20%), and fewer men than women disagreed (70% and 76%). (Both results statistically significant.) The percentage that agreed with the statement that getting HIV is something that worried them, was broken down by cluster group, significantly more people in cluster A (39%) agreed with the statement than people in cluster B (18%).

Figure 5.31 shows that there are significantly more people in cluster group A at higher or moderate risk in comparison to cluster B (7% and 3%; 5% and 3% respectively). Significantly more people in cluster group A correctly perceived their risk to be great or quite a lot in comparison to cluster group B (6% and 2%) (Figure 5.32).

Only 4% of men and 3% of women had sought voluntary testing for HIV, those seeking tests did not differ by risk group (Table 5.15).

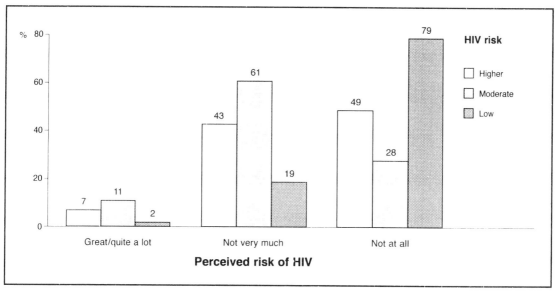

Chi-squared test for high risk compared with low risk p < 0.05 for each perceived risk

Fig. 5.30. Percentage distribution of perceived risk of HIV by computed risk of HIV

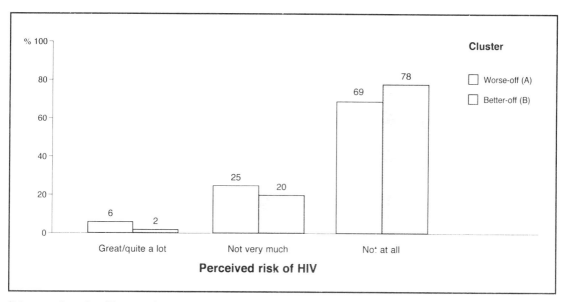

Chi-squared test for differences between clusters p < 0.05 for all

Fig. 5.31. Percentage distribution of perceived risk of HIV by cluster group

Discussion

As age at first intercourse is decreasing, particularly for those in manual occupations, and as contraception use is less likely at first intercourse for those in the 'worse-off' demographic cluster, there is a need to continue to emphasise safer sex messages in school education for those younger than 16 years of age. Sex education is clearly having an impact given that in fact very few people do not use any form of contraception when they first have sex. Most people support the inclusion of information about contraception in school sex education.

Women would like to see more inclusion of topics about feelings, emotions and personal choice. A substantial minority would wish to see information about homosexuality and lesbianism included. As most men and women think parents should be included in sex education there is a need to continue to develop sex education programmes that are sensitive to parents' wishes and involve them.

There was a clear indication that adverts about AIDS and condoms are socially acceptable and should be allowed to be screened before the 9 pm watershed.

There were low levels of knowledge about some significant sexual health risks. Respondents did not feel they had adequate knowledge about emergency contraception, recognising the symptoms of STDs, or having an HIV test. Given the concerns about the rates of teenage pregnancy, the wider provision of emergency contraception services and their advertisement is warranted. Consideration should also be given to the training needs of staff in doctors' surgeries, accident and emergency departments and others who may come in contact with pregnant young women. More information is also required about STD symptoms and when to visit the GP/GUM clinic.

There should be a more integrated approach to the provision of education about STDs. There is a need to understand more about why people stop using barrier methods and change to the pill. What are the determinants of continued condom use, or conversely cessation? What psychological factors are there in steady relationships that allow people to feel safe and able to stop using condoms, with no evidence as to the HIV status of their partners? Do men put pressure on women to go on the pill – if so why? What about the more recent scares about the long-term effects of the pill?

People not in steady relationships believed that 'getting carried away' would stop them using condoms, and often people said that they didn't use condoms because they forgot to carry them. There should be greater encouragement for those who are likely to need to use them and among those at highest risk, to carry condoms at all times. Research is required to establish whether making the carrying of condoms more socially acceptable, would encourage their use.

References

Wellings, K, Field, J, Johnson, A and Wadsworth, J with Bradshaw, S (1994). *Sexual behaviour in Britain: the National Survey of Sexual Attitudes and Lifestyles*. London: Penguin Books.

6. Association between nutrition, smoking and sexual health

Introduction

In this chapter the association between nutrition, smoking and sexual health is explored. The objective is to assess whether people who were at risk for one factor were also at risk for other factors. The cluster variables have been used to define the demographic, dietary and sexual health profiles of respondents.

Association between smoking and nutrition

- Smokers eat less healthily than never or ex-smokers.
- Smokers in the North and the Midlands eat less healthily than smokers in the South.
- Smokers in younger, low-income families and the older, less-educated group eat less healthily.
- There appears to be a relationship between smoking cessation and changing to a healthier diet.

Table 6.1 presents the proportion of respondents eating a more healthy diet by smoking status (as defined by cigarette smoking), for men and women separately.

Current smokers of either gender were less likely to be eating a more healthy diet than never smokers (men – current 33%, never 51%; women – current 46%, never 58%). For men, there was little difference in the proportion eating a more healthy diet among those who had never smoked. Among women who never smoked 58% were currently eating a healthy diet. Irrespective of smoking status women were more likely to be eating a more healthy diet than men (all gender differences statistically significant).

Generally about 39% of respondents who smoked ate a more healthy diet, whereas in Trent, West Midlands and the North-West regions 32% of smokers ate a more healthy diet compared with 51% in the North Thames region.

Table 6.1. Percentage distribution of more healthy dietary cluster by smoking status by gender

	Men More healthy (%)	Women More healthy (%)
Smoking status[1]		
Current	33	46
Ex-smoker	55	64
Never smoked	51	58
Base: all[2]		

[1]Chi-squared test between smoking status groups within gender p < 0.05 for all except between ex- and never smokers for men
[2]Missing 5% men and 4% women

The relationship between eating a healthy diet and smoking status was explored further within each demographic cluster (Figure 6.1). Within demographic clusters, that is controlling for demographic differences, never and ex-smokers were statistically significantly less likely to be eating a less healthy diet than smokers. Smokers in the younger, low-income families cluster and the older, less-educated group (clusters 2 and 4) were statistically

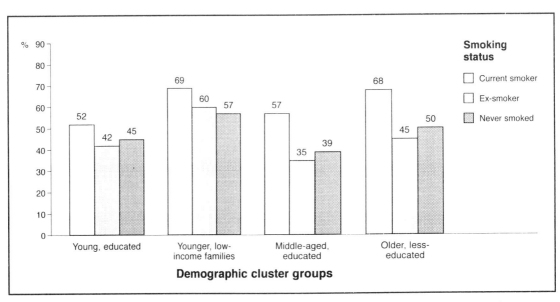

Chi-squared test for differences between current smoker and ex-smoker or never smoked p < 0.05 except for current smoker v. ex-smoker – younger, low-income families. No differences between ex- and never smoked

Fig. 6.1. Percentage of respondents eating a less healthy diet by smoking status and demographic cluster group

Table 6.2. Percentage distribution of dietary change by smoking status by gender

	Men[1]			Women[1]		
	Current smoker (%)	Ex-smoker (%)	Never smoked (%)	Current smoker (%)	Ex-smoker (%)	Never smoked
No dietary change	36	17	22 [abc]	23	12	14 [ab]
Already healthy	23	27	26 [a]	20	23	27
Other changes	7	12	8 [ab]	12	13	10 [c]
Changed to more healthy diet	37	53	50 [ab]	52	61	56 [ac]
Base:[2]						

[1]Chi-squared test for differences between smoking status groups $p < 0.05$ for [a]smokers versus ex-smokers, [b]smoker versus never smoked, [c]never smoked versus ex-smoker
[2]Missing 3% men and 2% women

significantly more likely to be eating a less healthy diet than smokers in the young educated and middle-aged educated clusters (1 and 3). These data suggest that, while the socio-demographic variables measured and included in the cluster analysis affected the relationship between smoking status and eating a more healthy diet, other factors must also be influencing the relationship beside variables included in the cluster analysis.

When subjects' responses to whether their diet has changed in the last three years were broken down by smoking status (Table 6.2) it was apparent that ex-smokers of either gender were more likely to have changed to a healthier diet (53% of men and 61% of women ex-smokers compared with 37% and 52% for current men and women smokers respectively, statistically significant within gender). Within each category of smoking, women were more likely to have changed to a more healthy diet than men. Over a third of male smokers had made no dietary change over the last three years, compared with 17% for male ex-smokers. It therefore seems that giving up smoking is associated with eating more healthily; this may indicate an awareness of risk and motivation to change lifestyle which affects more than one risk factor. It is not clear from these data whether change in one area preceded that in another; this would be an important area for further study which would influence practice in supporting health behaviour change.

The proportion of subjects in each smoking category who had made healthy changes to their diet over the last three years broken down by demographic clusters is presented in Figure 6.2. For each smoking category demographic clusters 1 and 3 were more likely to have made healthy changes to their diets than clusters 2 and 4; the group least likely to have changed their diets was smokers in cluster 4 (older less educated).

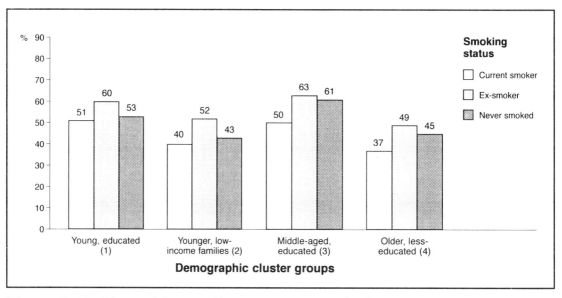

Chi-squared test for differences between smoking status groups p < 0.05 for all except:
cluster 1, smoker v. never smoked; cluster 2, never v. smoked or ex-smoker; clusters 3 and 4 ex- v. never smoked

Fig. 6.2. Percentage of respondents changing to a more healthy diet over the last three years by smoking status by demographic cluster group

Association between smoking and sexual health

• Smokers are more likely to have a higher HIV risk.

The sexual health risk score for respondents was broken down by current smoking status for respondents who had had sexual intercourse (Table 6.3). Respondents at lowest sexual health risk were less likely to be current smokers than those at moderate or higher risk (groups combined as numbers small and percentage distribution was the same, 30% compared with 48%).

Table 6.3. Percentage distribution of smoking status by HIV risk

	Higher/Moderate[1] (%)	Low[2] (%)
Current smoker	48	30
Ex-smoker	30	37
Never smoked	22	34
Base:[3]		

[1]Higher and moderate not combined as no difference between the groups across smoking categories
[2]Chi-squared test for higher/moderate versus low risk p < 0.05 for all
[3]Those who have had sexual intercourse (data for men and women combined). Missing 1% men and women

Association between nutrition and sexual health

> • People at lowest HIV risk are more likely to eat a more healthy diet.
> • People at highest HIV risk are less likely to change to a healthier diet.

Table 6.4 presents the distribution of respondents' dietary cluster group broken down by HIV risk group. Respondents at low HIV risk were more likely to be in the more healthy dietary cluster group than those at high risk (53% among low HIV risk, compared with 43% among higher HIV risk).

Table 6.4. Percentage distribution of dietary cluster by HIV risk group

| | HIV risk group[1] | | |
	Higher (%)	Moderate (%)	Low (%)
More healthy	43	50	53
Base:[2]			

[1] Chi-squared test for differences between HIV risk groups ($p < 0.05$)
[2] Those who have had sexual intercourse. Missing 2% men and 2% women

Because subjects over 55 years were not asked to complete the sexual health questionnaire the number of subjects in this analysis is reduced. The demographic cluster variable derived for all respondents was re-calculated because cluster 4 highlighted mainly older subjects. In the present analysis there are only two demographic clusters: a 'worse-off' cluster reflecting respondents who were in cluster 2, the 'younger, low-income and less-education group'; and effectively 1 and 3 from the larger sample demographic clusters being defined as one better educated and employed cluster, or 'better-off' cluster.

Respondents classified at moderate or higher HIV risk were more likely to have not changed their diet over the last three years compared with those respondents at low risk (higher or moderate risk, no dietary change – 25%; low risk, no change – 19%). There was little difference in the proportion of respondents changing to a more healthy diet between health risk groups. Sixty-one per cent of men and 53% of women in the higher risk group were currently eating a less healthy diet compared with 52% for men and 43% for women in the lowest risk category.

Table 6.5 explored whether there was any association between cost limitations for choosing a healthy diet and the use of condoms broken down by demographic cluster. Respondents in the younger low-income families (worse-off cluster) were more likely to agree that healthy eating was expensive and that cost was a factor in determining the use of condoms (22% in worse-off cluster compared with 10% in better-off cluster).

Table 6.5. Percentage distribution of respondents considering healthy food is expensive with the proportion of respondents reporting that the cost of condoms as a likely cause of not using condoms by cluster groups

The cost of condoms as a cause of not using condoms	Agree healthy food is expensive (%)	
	Worse-off cluster[1]	Better-off cluster
Unlikely	78	90
Likely	22	10
Base:[2]		

[1]Chi-squared test for differences between clusters p < 0.05 for all
[2]Those who have had sexual intercourse. Missing 18% respondents

Association between smoking, nutrition and sexual health

- Ex- and never smokers at low HIV risk were more likely to eat a healthy diet than current smokers at higher HIV risk.

The percentage of subjects eating a more healthy diet was broken down by sexual health risk and smoking status (Table 6.6).

The number of respondents in this analysis is small and differences between groups are not statistically significant. The data suggest, however, that ex- and never smokers at low risk of HIV were more likely to be eating a healthy diet than current smokers at higher HIV risk.

Table 6.6. Percentage distribution of respondents eating a more healthy diet (dietary cluster) by HIV risk by smoking status

	More healthy diet[1]	
	Higher and moderate risk of HIV	Low risk of HIV
Smoking status[1]	%	%
Current smoker	42	39
Ex-smoker	53	59
Never smoker	46	59
Base:[2]		

[1]Chi-squared test for differences within smoking status groups between HIV risk and dietary cluster groups none statistically significant p < 0.05
[2]Base: those who have had sexual intercourse. Missing 14%

Discussion

This study has shown clear associations between nutrition, smoking and sexual behaviour. Those people who smoke are likely to have the poorest diet and the highest sexual risk. The cluster analyses showed that those people who were from younger, low-income families or older less-educated groups were more likely to have the highest rates of smoking, sexual health risk and to be eating a less healthy diet. Targeting health promotion activity at the more vulnerable sections of the population would reach those at most health risk. Particularly vulnerable groups are the elderly, those on low income and single parents which are represented by the clusters seen to be at most risk by this analysis.

The recognition that smokers have excess risk from eating less healthy diets indicates that attention should be paid to their nutritional status alongside support to motivate smoking cessation. The positive associations seen between changing to a healthier diet and giving up smoking suggest that motivation to change health risk behaviour may generalise between behaviours. Understanding more about the relationships between change in different aspects of lifestyle in order to encourage and support health behaviour change over the longer term would contribute to more sensitive and effective health promotion interventions, particularly with those sections of the population who are at multiple health risk.

Appendices

Appendix A. Questionnaire

HEALTH AND LIFESTYLE SURVEY 1993

Good morning, etc. I'm ... from MORI. We are carrying out a survey on behalf of the Health Education Authority, about the health and lifestyle of people living in Britain today. But before I start asking you specifically about health, I wonder if I could ask a few more general questions about yourself and your household. Everything you tell me is totally confidential.

STICK ADDRESS NUMBER LABEL IN THIS SPACE

(11-16)

CODE DAY OF WEEK OF INTERVIEW

	(17)
Monday	1
Tuesday	2
Wednesday	3
Thursday	4
Friday	5
Saturday	6
Sunday	7

(17)

INTERVIEWER DECLARATION

I confirm that I have conducted this interview face-to-face with the person named on the contact sheet for this address and that I asked all the relevant questions and recorded the answers in conformance with the survey specifications and within the MRS Code of Conduct.

DATE OF INTERVIEW . . . .

INTERVIEWER NAME . . . .

SIGNATURE . . . .

INTERVIEWER NUMBER ☐ ☐ ☐ ☐ / ☐

               (18) (19) (20) (21)   (22)

(18-22)

DEMOGRAPHICS

Q1   **How many people are there usually living here in this household - that includes yourself, any other adults and children?**

NB INCLUDE THOSE 75+   ☐☐   people

(23)(24)   (23-24)

ASK IF MORE THAN ONE PERSON IN HH (IF ONE, GO TO Q3)

Q2   **What relationship is each person to you?**
RESPONDENT IS ALWAYS PERSON 1 FROM NOW ON
CODE BELOW RELATIONSHIP TO RESPONDENT FOR EACH PERSON
IF MORE THAN 6 PEOPLE USE CONTINUATION SHEET

	Person 1	Person 2 (25)	Person 3 (27)	Person 4 (29)	Person 5 (31)	Person 6 (33)
Respondent	1					
Spouse		2	2	2	2	2
Partner		3	3	3	3	3
Daughter/son		4	4	4	4	4
Daughter-in-law/son-in-law		5	5	5	5	5
Child of spouse/partner		6	6	6	6	6
Father/mother		7	7	7	7	7
Father-in-law/mother-in-law		8	8	8	8	8
Stepfather/stepmother		9	9	9	9	9
Grandparent/in-law		0	0	0	0	0
Grandchild (inc step)		X	X	X	X	X
Brother/sister (inc step)		Y	Y	Y	Y	Y
		(26)	(28)	(30)	(32)	(34)
Aunt/uncle (inc step)		1	1	1	1	1
Nephew/niece/in-law		2	2	2	2	2
Cousin/in-law (inc step)		3	3	3	3	3
Other relation (by blood, marriage or adoption)		4	4	4	4	4
Lodger		5	5	5	5	5
Unrelated sharer/flatmate		6	6	6	6	6
Other (WRITE IN & CODE 7)	7					

. . . . 7

. . . . 7

. . . . 7

. . . . 7   (25-34)

Q3   RECORD EACH PERSON'S GENDER

	Person 1 (35)	Person 2 (36)	Person 3 (37)	Person 4 (38)	Person 5 (39)	Person 6 (40)
Female	1	1	1	1	1	1
Male	2	2	2	2	2	2

(35-40)

Q4   **And how old are you? How old is he/she?** ENTER FOR EACH PERSON IN BOXES BELOW
FOR BABIES LESS THAN 12 MONTHS OLD, ENTER "00"

Person 1	Person 2	Person 3	Person 4	Person 5	Person 6
☐☐	☐☐	☐☐	☐☐	☐☐	☐☐
(41) (42)	(43) (44)	(45) (46)	(47) (48)	(49) (50)	(51) (52)

(41-52)

Q5   SHOWCARD A (R)   **Which statement on this card applies to you/him/her?**

		Respondent Person 1 (53)	Person 2 (55)	Person 3 (57)	Person 4 (59)	Person 5 (61)	Person 6 (63)
1.	Paid employee working full-time (30+ hrs/week)	1	1	1	1	1	1
2.	Paid employee working part-time (up to 29hrs/week)	2	2	2	2	2	2
3.	Self-employed working full-time	3	3	3	3	3	3
4.	Self-employed working part-time	4	4	4	4	4	4
5.	Retired with occupational pension	5	5	5	5	5	5
6.	Retired on state benefits only	6	6	6	6	6	6
7.	Unemployed for less than 6 months	7	7	7	7	7	7
8.	Unemployed for more than 6 months	8	8	8	8	8	8
9.	Waiting to take up a job already obtained	9	9	9	9	9	9
10.	Temporarily sick/disabled less than 6 months	0	0	0	0	0	0
11.	Long term sick/disabled (6 months or longer)	X	X	X	X	X	X
12.	On government training scheme	Y	Y	Y	Y	Y	Y
		(54)	(56)	(58)	(60)	(62)	(64)
13.	Looking after home or family	1	1	1	1	1	1
14.	Pre-school		2	2	2	2	2
15.	At school	3	3	3	3	3	3
16.	Other full-time education	4	4	4	4	4	4

(53-64)

ASK IF MORE THAN ONE PERSON IN HH (IF ONE, CIRCLE CODE 1)

Q6   **Can I check which person is the head of the household? This means the person who owns or rents the household's accommodation** PROBE AS NECESSARY, USE STANDARD RULES FOR DEFINITION OF HOH. CIRCLE PERSON NUMBER

Person Number   1   2   3   4   5   6   7   8   9 _____ (65)

NOW FOLLOW ROUTING BELOW IN COLUMN FOR RESPONDENT

EMPLOYMENT STATUS AT Q5	RESPONDENT	SPOUSE/PARTNER	HEAD OF HOUSEHOLD (IF NOT RESP OR PARTNER)
IF NO. 1, 2, 3, 4	ASK Q7a	Q25a	Q43a
IF NO. 5, 6	GOTO Q19a	Q37a	Q55a
IF NO. 7, 8, 9	GOTO Q16	Q34	Q52
IF NO. 10, 11, 13	GOTO Q18	Q36	Q54
IF NO. 12	ASK Q7a	Q25a	Q43a
IF NO. 15, 16	GOTO Q10	Q28	Q46

RESPONDENT (PERSON 1)

Q7a ASK IF NOS. 1-4 (WORKING FULL OR PART-TIME) OR 12 (GOVT SCHEME) AT Q5
What is the name or title of your job? PROBE FOR GRADE IF NECESSARY

. . . .

Q7b **What industry do you work in?**

. . . .

Q7c **What kind of work do you do most of the time?**

. . . .

Q7d **Do you have any special training or qualifications for that job, or do you use any machinery or special skills?**

. . . .
. . . .
. . . .

Q8a ASK IF NOS 1-2 (EMPLOYEE) or 12 (GOVT SCHEME) AT Q5
Are you a manager or a foreman or supervisor, or not?

(66)
Manager 1
Foreman/supervisor 2
Other type of employee 3

Q8b **How many employees work in the establishment?**

1-2 4
3-24 5
25-99 6
100-999 7
1000 or more 8   (66)
(IF GOVERNMENT SCHEME AT Q5, NOW GOTO Q18. OTHERS NOW GOTO P7)

Q9 ASK IF NOS 3-4 (SELF-EMPLOYED) AT Q5
Do you employ any other people? How many?

(67)
1-5 employees 1
6-24 employees 2
25 or more employees 3
No employees 4   (67)
(IF GOVERNMENT SCHEME AT Q5, NOW GOTO Q18. OTHERS GOTO P7)

Q10 ASK IF NOS 15/16 (SCHOOL/OTHER FULL-TIME EDUCATION) AT Q5
Can I just check, are you in any paid job or doing any paid work at the moment?

	(68)		
Yes	1	ASK Q11	
No	2	GOTO P7	(68)

Q11a ASK IF YES AT Q10 (IF NO, SEE Q25a)
What is the name or title of your job? PROBE GRADE

. . . .

Q11b **What industry do you work in?**

. . . .

Q11c **What kind of work do you do most of the time?**

. . . .

Q11d **Do you have any special training or qualifications for that job, or do you use any machinery or special skills?**

. . . .

. . . .

Q12 **Are you an employee or self-employed?**

	(69)	
Employee	1	
Self-employed	2	(69)

Q13 **How many hours a week do you usually work?**

☐☐ hours
(70) (71)   (70-71)

Q14a ASK IF EMPLOYEE AT Q12
Are you a manager or a foreman or supervisor, or not?

	(72)
Manager	1
Foreman/supervisor	2
Other type of employee	3

Q14b **How many employees work in the establishment?**

1-2	4	
3-24	5	
25-99	6	
100-999	7	
1000 or more	8	NOW GO TO P7 (72)

ASK IF SELF-EMPLOYED AT Q12
Q15   **Do you employ any other people? How many?**

                                                    (73)

1-5 employees 1
6-24 employees 2
25 or more employees 3
None 4   NOW GO TO P7 (73)

ASK IF NOS 7, 8, 9 (UNEMPLOYED/WAITING TO TAKE UP JOB) AT Q5
Q16   **How long altogether have you been out of employment but wanting work, in this current period of unemployment (that is, since any time you may have spent on a government scheme such as YTS or ET)?**

(74)

Less than 1 week 1
1 week but less than 1 month 2
1 months but less than 3 months 3
3 months but less than 6 months 4
6 months but less than 12 months 5
12 months but less than 2 years 6
2 years but less than 3 years 7
3 years but less than 5 years 8
5 years or more 9 (74)

ASK IF No. 9 (WAITING TO TAKE UP A JOB) AT Q5
Q17   **Apart from the job you are waiting to take up, have you ever had a paid job or done any paid work?**

(75)

Yes ..... 1 ASK Q19a
No ..... 2 GOTO P7 (75)

ASK IF NOS 7, 8, 10, 11, 12, 13 AT Q5
Q18   **Have you ever had a paid job or done any paid work?**

(76)

Yes ..... 1 ASK Q19a
No ..... 2 GOTO P7 (76)

ASK IF YES AT Q17 OR Q18, OR IF NOS 5-6 AT Q5 (RETIRED)
Q19a **In your last paid job or paid work, what was the name or title of your job?** (PROBE GRADE IF NECESSARY)

....

Q19b **What industry did you work in?**

....

Q19c **What kind of work did you do most of the time?**

....

Q19d **Did you have any special training or qualifications for that job, or did you use any machinery or special skills?**

....
....

Q20 **Did you work full-time or part-time?**

(77)
Full-time (30+ hrs/week) 1
Part-time (8 up to 29 hrs/week) 2   (77)

Q21 **Were you an employee or self-employed?**

(78)
Employee 1   ASK Q22
Self-employed 2   GOTO Q23   (78)

ASK IF EMPLOYEE AT Q21
Q22a **Were you a manager or a foreman or supervisor, or not?**

(79)
Manager 1
Foreman/supervisor 2
Other type of employee 3   (79)

Q22b **How many employees worked in the establishment?**

(80)
1-2 . . . . 1 ⎤
3-24 . . . . 2 ⎥
25-99 . . . . 3 ⎬
100-999 . . . . 4 ⎥
1000 or more . . . . 5 ⎦   NOW SEE Q24   (80)

CARD ② 10

ASK IF SELF-EMPLOYED AT Q21
Q23 **Did you employ any other people? How many?**

(11)
1-5 employees . . . . 1 ⎤
6-24 employees . . . . 2 ⎬
25 or more employees . . . . 3 ⎥
No employees . . . . 4 ⎦   NOW SEE Q24   (11)

ASK IF RETIRED (NOS 5 OR 6) AT Q5
Q24 **At what age did you retire?**

☐ ☐ years
(12)   (13)

(12-13)

(14-19)

RESPONDENT'S SPOUSE/PARTNER

INTERVIEWER CHECK:

No spouse/partner in HH at Q2 1   GO TO P11
Spouse/partner in HH recorded at Q2 2   ASK Q25 ETC

CHECK BACK TO BOX ON P2 FOR ROUTING

Now I'd like to ask some questions about your husband/wife/partner

ASK IF NOS. 1-4 (WORKING FULL OR PART-TIME) OR 12 (GOVT SCHEME) AT Q5
Q25a **What is the name or title of his/her job? PROBE FOR GRADE IF NECESSARY**

....

Q25b **What industry does he/she work in?**

....

Q25c **What kind of work does he/she do most of the time?**

....

Q25d **Does he/she have any special training or qualifications for that job, or does he/she use any machinery or special skills?**

....

....

ASK IF NOS 1-2 (EMPLOYEE) or 12 (GOVT SCHEME) AT Q5
Q26a **Is he/she a manager or a foreman or supervisor, or not?**

(20)
Manager 1
Foreman/supervisor 2
Other type of employee 3   (20)

Q26b **How many employees work in the establishment?**

(21)
1-2 1
3-24 2
25-99 3
100-999 4
1000 or more 5
(IF GOVT SCHEME AT Q5, NOW GOTO Q36. OTHERS NOW GOTO P11)   (21)

ASK IF NOS 3-4 (SELF-EMPLOYED) AT Q5
Q27 **Does he/she employ any other people? How many?**

(22)
1-5 employees 1
6-24 employees 2
25 or more employees 3
No employees 4
(IF GOVT SCHEME AT Q5, NOW GOTO Q36. OTHERS NOW GOTO P11)   (22)

8

ASK IF NOS 15/16 (SCHOOL/OTHER FULL-TIME EDUCATION) AT Q5
Q28   **Can I just check, is he/she in any paid job or doing any paid work at the moment?**

                                                                    (23)
          Yes 1   ASK Q29 ETC
          No 2   GOTO P11   (23)

ASK IF YES
Q29a   **What is the name or title of his/her job? PROBE GRADE**

          . . . .

Q29b   **What industry does he/she work in?**

          . . . .

Q29c   **What kind of work does he/she do most of the time?**

          . . . .

Q29d   **Does he/she have any special training or qualifications for that job, or does he/she use any machinery or special skills?**

          . . . .
          . . . .

Q30   **Is he/she an employee or self-employed?**

                                                                    (23)
          Employee 3
          Self-employed 4   (23)

Q31   **How many hours a week does he/she usually work?**

          ☐☐ hours
          (24) (25)   (24-25)

ASK IF EMPLOYEE AT Q30
Q32a   **Is he/she a manager or a foreman or supervisor, or not?**

                                                                    (26)
          Manager 1
          Foreman/supervisor 2
          Other type of employee 3

Q32b   **How many employees work in the establishment?**

          1-2 4
          3-24 5
          25-99 6
          100-999 7
          1000 or more 8   NOW GO TO P11 (26)

ASK IF SELF-EMPLOYED AT Q30
Q33 **Does he/she employ any other people? How many?**

<pre>
                                                         (27)
     1-5 employees 1
     6-24 employees 2
     25 or more employees 3
     None 4   NOW GO TO P11 (27)
</pre>

ASK IF NOS 7, 8, 9 (UNEMPLOYED/WAITING TO TAKE UP JOB) AT Q5
Q34 **How long altogether has he/she been out of employment but wanting work, in this current period of unemployment (that is, since any time he/she may have spent on a government scheme such as YTS or ET)?**

<pre>
                                                         (28)
     Less than 1 week 1
     1 week but less than 1 month 2
     1 months but less than 3 months 3
     3 months but less than 6 months 4
     6 months but less than 12 months 5
     12 months but less than 2 years 6
     2 years but less than 3 years 7
     3 years but less than 5 years 8
     5 years or more 9   (28)
</pre>

ASK IF NO. 9 (WAITING TO TAKE UP A JOB) AT Q5
Q35 **Apart from the job he/she is waiting to take up, has he/she ever had a paid job or done any paid work?**

<pre>
                                                         (29)
     Yes 1   ASK Q37a
     No 2   GOTO P11   (29)
</pre>

ASK IF NOS 7, 8, 10, 11, 12, 13 AT Q5
Q36 **Has he/she ever had a paid job or done any paid work?**

<pre>
                                                         (30)
     Yes 1   ASK Q37a
     No 2   GOTO P11   (30)
</pre>

ASK IF YES AT Q35 OR Q36, OR IF NOS 5-6 AT Q5 (RETIRED)
Q37a **In his/her last paid job or paid work, what was the name or title of his/her job?** (PROBE GRADE IF NECESSARY)

....

Q37b **What industry did he/she work in?**

....

Q37c **What kind of work did he/she do most of the time?**

....

Q37d **Did he/she have any special training or qualifications for that job, or did he/she use any machinery or special skills?**

....

....

Q38   **Did he/she work full-time or part-time?**

                                                                    (31)
            Full-time (30+ hrs/week) 1
            Part-time (8 up to 29 hrs/week) 2   (31)

Q39   **Was he/she an employee or self-employed?**

                                                                    (32)
            Employee 1   ASK Q40
            Self-employed 2   GOTO Q41   (32)

        ASK IF EMPLOYEE AT Q39
Q40a   **Was he/she a manager or a foreman or supervisor, or not?**

                                                                    (33)
            Manager 1
            Foreman/supervisor 2
            Other type of employee 3   (33)

Q40b   **How many employees worked in the establishment?**

                                                                    (34)
            1-2 . . . . 1 ⎫
            3-24 . . . . 2 ⎬
            25-99 . . . . 3 ⎬
            100-999 . . . . 4 ⎬
            1000 or more . . . . 5 ⎭   NOW SEE Q42   (34)

        ASK IF SELF-EMPLOYED AT Q39
Q41   **Did he/she employ any other people? How many?**

                                                                    (35)
            1-5 employees . . . . 1 ⎫
            6-24 employees . . . . 2 ⎬
            25 or more employees . . . . 3 ⎬
            No employees . . . . 4 ⎭   NOW SEE Q42   (35)

        ASK IF RETIRED (NOS 5 OR 6) AT Q5
Q42   **At what age did he/she retire?**

            ☐ ☐ years
            (36) (37)   (36-37)

                                                                                 (38-43)

HEAD OF HOUSEHOLD

INTERVIEWER CHECK:

RESPONDENT IS HOH AT Q6	1	SEE Q61
SPOUSE/PARTNER IS HOH AT Q6	2	GO TO Q62
OTHER PERSON IS HOH AT Q6	3	ASK Q43 etc

(CHECK BOX ON P2 FOR ROUTING)

Now I'd like to ask some questions about the head of your household.

ASK IF NOS. 1-4 (WORKING FULL OR PART-TIME) OR 12 (GOVT SCHEME) AT Q5
Q43a   **What is the name or title of his/her job? PROBE FOR GRADE IF NECESSARY**

. . . .

Q43b   **What industry does he/she work in?**

. . . .

Q43c   **What kind of work does he/she do most of the time?**

. . . .

Q43d   **Does he/she have any special training or qualifications for that job, or does he/she use any machinery or special skills?**

. . . .

. . . .

ASK IF NOS 1-2 (EMPLOYEE) or 12 (GOVT SCHEME) AT Q5
Q44a   **Is he/she a manager or a foreman or supervisor, or not?**

	(44)	
Manager	1	
Foreman/supervisor	2	
Other type of employee	3	(44)

Q44b   **How many employees work in the establishment?**

	(45)	
1-2	1	
3-24	2	
25-99	3	
100-999	4	
1000 or more	5	(45)

(IF GOVT SCHEME AT Q5, NOW GOTO Q54. OTHERS SEE Q61)

ASK IF NOS 3-4 (SELF-EMPLOYED) AT Q5
Q45   **Does he/she employ any other people? How many?**

	(46)	
1-5 employees	1	
6-24 employees	2	
25 or more employees	3	
No employees	4	(46)

(IF GOVT SCHEME AT Q5, NOW GOTO Q54. OTHERS SEE Q61)

ASK IF NOS 15/16 (SCHOOL/OTHER FULL-TIME EDUCATION) AT Q5
Q46   **Can I just check, is he/she in any paid job or doing any paid work at the moment?**

(47)
Yes 1   ASK Q47 etc
No 2   SEE Q61   (47)

ASK IF YES
Q47a   **What is the name or title of his/her job?**   PROBE GRADE

. . . .

Q47b   **What industry does he/she work in?**

. . . .

Q47c   **What kind of work does he/she do most of the time?**

. . . .

Q47d   **Does he/she have any special training or qualifications for that job, or does he/she use any machinery or special skills?**

. . . .

. . . .

Q48   **Is he/she an employee or self-employed?**

(47)
Employee 3
Self-employed 4   (47)

Q49   **How many hours a week does he/she usually work?**

☐☐ hours
(48)   (49)   (48-49)

ASK IF EMPLOYEE AT Q48
Q50a   **Is he/she a manager or a foreman or supervisor, or not?**

(50)
Manager 1
Foreman/supervisor 2
Other type of employee 3   (50)

Q50b   **How many employees work in the establishment?**

(50)
1-2 4
3-24 5
25-99 6
100-999 7
1000 or more 8   NOW SEE Q61   (50)

ASK IF SELF-EMPLOYED AT Q48
Q51   **Does he/she employ any other people? How many?**

(51)
1-5 employees 1
6-24 employees 2
25 or more employees 3
None 4   NOW SEE Q61   (51)

Q52 ASK IF NOS 7, 8, 9 (UNEMPLOYED/WAITING TO TAKE UP JOB) AT Q5
How long altogether has he/she been out of employment but wanting work, in this current period of unemployment (that is, since any time he/she may have spent on a government scheme such as YTS or ET)?

	(52)
Less than 1 week	1
1 week but less than 1 month	2
1 months but less than 3 months	3
3 months but less than 6 months	4
6 months but less than 12 months	5
12 months but less than 2 years	6
2 years but less than 3 years	7
3 years but less than 5 years	8
5 years or more	9

(52)

Q53 ASK IF NO. 9 (WAITING TO TAKE UP A JOB) AT Q5
Apart from the job he/she is waiting to take up, has he/she ever had a paid job or done any paid work?

	(53)	
Yes	1	ASK Q55
No	2	SEE Q61

(53)

Q54 ASK IF NOS 7, 8, 10, 11, 12, 13 AT Q5
Has he/she ever had a paid job or done any paid work?

	(54)	
Yes	1	ASK Q55
No	2	SEE Q61

(54)

Q55a ASK IF YES AT Q53 OR Q54, OR IF NOS 5-6 AT Q5 (RETIRED)
In his/her last paid job or paid work, what was the name or title of his/her job? (PROBE GRADE IF NECESSARY)

. . . .

Q55b **What industry did he/she work in?**

. . . .

Q55c **What kind of work did he/she do most of the time?**

. . . .

Q55d **Did he/she have any special training or qualifications for that job, or did he/she use any machinery or special skills?**

. . . .

. . . .

Q56 **Did he/she work full-time or part-time?**

	(55)
Full-time (30+ hrs/week)	1
Part-time (8 up to 29 hrs/week)	2

(55)

Q57 **Was he/she an employee or self-employed?**

	(56)	
Employee	1	ASK Q58
Self-employed	2	GOTO Q59

(56)

ASK IF EMPLOYEE AT Q57

Q58a **Was he/she a manager or a foreman or supervisor, or not?**

	(57)
Manager	1
Foreman/supervisor	2
Other type of employee	3	(57)

Q58b **How many employees worked in the establishment?**

	(58)
1-2	1
3-24	2
25-99	3
100-999	4
1000 or more	5	NOW SEE Q60 (58)

ASK IF SELF-EMPLOYED AT Q57

Q59 **Did he/she employ any other people? How many?**

	(59)
1-5 employees	1
6-24 employees	2
25 or more employees	3
No employees	4	NOW SEE Q60 (59)

ASK IF RETIRED (NOS 5 OR 6) AT Q5

Q60 **At what age did he/she retire?**

☐☐ years
(60) (61)   (60-61)

                                                                    (62-67)

ASK IF RESPONDENT HAS <u>NO</u> SPOUSE/PARTNER IN HOUSEHOLD AT Q2 (OTHERS ASK Q62)

Q61 **Can you tell me please what is your own total income? This is your personal income from all sources, before tax and other deductions. (It also includes money from part-time or temporary jobs, pocket money, allowances or student grants.)**
Please include all benefits, such as child benefit, Income Support, retirement pensions, or unemployment benefit. ENTER IN BOXES TO NEAREST £

£ ☐☐☐ , ☐☐☐
(68) (69) (70)   (71) (72) (73)

Don't know	X	
Refused	Y	ASK Q64	(68-73)

ASK IF RESPONDENT HAS SPOUSE/PARTNER IN HOUSEHOLD AT Q2

Q62 **Can you tell me please what is the total income of yourself and your husband/wife/partner? This is your income from all sources, before tax and other deductions. (It also includes money from part-time or temporary jobs, pocket money, allowances or student grants.) Please include all benefits such as child benefit, Income Support, retirement pensions or unemployment benefit.**
ENTER IN BOXES TO NEAREST £

£ ☐☐☐ , ☐☐☐
(74) (75) (76)   (77) (78) (79)

Don't know	X	
Refused	Y	ASK Q64	(74-79)

CARD③   10

INTERVIEWER PLEASE RECORD FOR ALL EXCEPT DON'T KNOW/REFUSED AT Q61 OR 62 (ASK IF NECESSARY)

Q63 **And is this per year, per month or per week?**

	(11)
Year	1
Month	2
Week	3	(11)

15

ASK IF DON'T KNOW/REFUSED AT Q61 OR Q62 (OTHERS GOTO Q65)

Q64 SHOWCARD B **Could you give me a letter from this card for the range in which you would put your total income? Again, I mean your (and your husband's/wife's/partner's) income from all sources, before tax and other deduction. (Please include money from part-time or temporary jobs, pocket money, allowances or student grants.) Please include all benefits, such as child benefit, income support, retirement pensions or unemployment benefit.**

	(12)
A	1
B	2
C	3
D	4
E	5
F	6
G	7
H	8
I	9
J	0
K	X
L	Y
	(13)
M	1
Don't know	2
Refused	3 (12-13)

ASK ALL

Q65 SHOWCARD C (R) **Do you (and your husband/wife/partner) receive any of these benefits?**

ASK IF OTHER ADULTS IN HH APART FROM RESPONDENT (AND PARTNER)

Q66 SHOWCARD C (R) AGAIN **Does any other person in your household receive any of these benefits?**

	Q65 (14)	Q66 (16)
Child benefit	1	1
State retirement pension	2	2
Income Support/social security	3	3
Unemployment benefit	4	4
Family Credit	5	5
Housing Benefit	6	6
Attendance Allowance	7	7
Invalid Care Allowance	8	8
Mobility Allowance	9	9
Sickness Benefit	0	0
Disablement living allowance	X	X
Invalidity pension/benefit or allowance	Y	Y
	(15)	(17)
Severe disablement benefit	1	1
Industrial disablement benefit	2	2
Maternity allowance	3	3
Other (WRITE IN & CODE '4')		
	4	4
None of these	5	5
Don't know	6	6 (14-17)

ASK ALL

Q67 SHOWCARD D   **Please look at this card and tell me which, if any, is the highest educational qualification you have obtained?**

(18)

A	CSE/GCE 'O' level/GCSE/Scottish 'O' Grade/ Scottish Standard Grade	1
B	GCE 'A' level/Scottish Higher Grade/Scottish Certificate of Sixth Year Studies (CSYS)	2
C	Recognised trade apprenticeship completed	3
D	Clerical and commercial qualifications (eg typing/ shorthand/book-keeping/commerce)	4
E	City and Guilds Certificate - Operative	5
F	City and Guilds Certificate - Craft/Intermediate/ Ordinary/Part 1	6
G	City and Guilds Certificate - Advanced/Final/Part II	7
H	City and Guilds - Full Technological(FTC)/Part III	8
I	Insignia Award in Technology (GCIA)	9
J	JIB/NHC or other Craft Technician Certificate	0
K	ONC/OND (or SNC/SND) or TEC/BEC/BTEC (or SCOTEC/SCOBEC/ SCOTVEC) National/General Certificate or Diploma	X
L	HNC/HND (or SHNC/SHND) or TEC/BEC/BTEC (or SCOTEC/ SCOBEC/SCOTVEC) Higher or Higher Cert or Diploma	Y

(19)

M	Nursing qualifications (eg SEN, SRN, SCM) - including Nursery Nursing (NNEC)	1
N	Polytechnic (or Central Institute) Diploma or Certificate (NOT CNAA VALIDATED)	2
O	University or CNAA Diploma or Certificate - including DIP HE and Teaching Training College Certificate	3
P	University or CNAA First Degree - including B Ed	4
Q	University or CNAA Post Graduate Diploma	5
R	University or CNAA Higher Degree - MSc, PhD, etc	6
S	Professional qualification - membership awarded by professional Institution	7
T	Any other qualification (WRITE IN & CODE '8')	
	....	8
U	No formal qualifications	9
V	Still studying - no qualifications yet	0
	Don't know	X (18-19)

Q68 SHOWCARD E   **Which of the statements on this card best describes you?**

(20)

1	Married	1
2	Single	2
3	Living with partner	3
4	Separated	4
5	Divorced	5
6	Widowed	6 (20)

Q69 **Does this household own this accommodation or do you rent it?** IF OWNED, PROBE TO FIND OUT IF CODE 1, 2 OR 3

(21)

Owned outright	1
Owned/being bought on mortgage	2
Bought from Council/under Right-to-Buy	3
Rented from Council	4
Rented from housing association	5
Rented from private landlord	6
Other (WRITE IN & CODE '7')	
....	7 (21)

Q70 **Does your household have the use of a telephone, or not?**

(22)

Yes	1
No	2 (22)

Q71 Now I'd like to ask some more detailed questions about your household's accommodation excluding any rooms you may let or sub-let. First of all, how many bed rooms does this accommodation have? IF BEDSIT, ENTER '01'

☐☐ bedrooms

Refused X   (23-24)

Q72 And how many living rooms does this accommodation have? IF BEDSIT, ENTER '00'

☐☐ livingrooms

Refused X   (25-26)

Q73 Does this accommodation have a bathroom which is for your household's use only?

	(27)
Yes 1	
No 2	
Refused 3	(27)

Q74 SHOWCARD F **What forms of heating do you use regularly in cold weather?** MULTICODE OK

(28)
Central heating:

Main gas 1		
Bottled gas 2		
Fuel oil 3		
Electricity	- normal tariff 4	
	- off peak 5	
Solid fuel	- smokeless 6	
	- non-smokeless 7	

Non-central heating:

Main gas fire/convector 8
Fan heaters 9
Electric bar fires 0
Storage heaters X
Calor/Butane gas heaters . . . . Y
(29)
Paraffin heaters 1
Oil filled electric radiator 2
Solid fuel open grate 3
Solid fuel stove/enclosed grate 4

Other (WRITE IN & CODE '5')

. . . . 5

Don't know 6   (28-29)

INTERVIEWER ASK OR CODE BY OBSERVATION
Q75 Address is:

(30)

House/bungalow:

- detached 1
- semi-detached 2
- Terraced/end of terrace 3

Maisonette 4
Flat 5
Rooms/bedsitter 6
Other (WRITE IN & CODE '7')

. . . . 7   (30)

Q76 Front door is on:

(31)

Basement 1
Ground floor/street level 2
1st floor 3
2nd floor 4
3rd floor 5
4th to 6th floor 6
7th to 9th floor 7
10th floor or higher 8   (31)

ASK ALL
Q77 **Do you own a car or have use of a car or van?**

(32)

Own car 1
Use of car (eg company car) 2
No car 3   (32)

Q78 **And do you personally have a full driver's licence, or not?**

(33)

Yes 1
No 2   (33)

Q79 **SHOWCARD G   From this card, which of these best describes your ethnic group?**

(34)

White 1
Black-Caribbean 2
Black-African 3
Black-Other (WRITE IN & CODE '4')

. . . . 4

Indian 5
Pakistani 6
Bangladeshi 7
Chinese 8
Any other ethnic group (WRITE IN & CODE '9')

. . . . 9   (34)

Q80   **Is English your first or main language?**

(35)

Yes 1

No 2   (35)

Q81   **In what country were you born?**

(36)

England 1

Scotland 2

Wales 3

N Ireland 4

Irish Republic (Eire) 5

West Indies/Guyana 6

India 7

Pakistan 8

Bangladesh 9

Other Asia (WRITE IN & CODE '0')

.... 0

Africa (WRITE IN AND CODE 'X')

.... X

Other country (WRITE IN & CODE 'Y')

.... Y   (36)

Q82   **Now, I would like to ask you some questions about your health in general. How do you feel about your health? Would you say that for your age your health is ...** READ OUT. ALTERNATE ORDER. TICK START

(37)

☐   **Very good** 1

Fairly good 2

Fairly poor 3

☐   **Very poor** 4

Don't know 5   (37)

Q83   **Do you have any long-standing illness, disability or infirmity? By long standing I mean anything that has troubled you over a period of time or that is likely to affect you over a period of time.**

(38)

Yes 1   ASK Q84

No 2   GO TO Q85   (38)

ASK IF YES AT Q83 (IF NO, GO TO Q85)

Q84   (a)   **What is the matter with you?** PROBE IN DETAIL **What else?** IF UNCLEAR ASK: **What do you mean by that?** WRITE IN

.... (39-40)

.... (41-42)

.... (43-44)

.... (45-46)

.... (47-48)

.... (49-50)

.... (51-52)

.... (53-54)

(b)   **Does this illness or disability (Do any of these illnesses or disabilities) limit your activities in any way?**

                                                             (55)

Yes 1
No 2   (55)

ASK ALL

Q85   SHOWCARD H (R)   This card list a number of things which may have happened to you. Could you tell me please which, if any, of these have happened to you in the past 12 months? You can just call out the number.

(56)

1 Serious illness or injury 1
2 Serious illness or injury of someone close to you 2
3 Death of a close relative or friend 3
4 Problems at work 4
5 Losing your job 5
6 Another member of this household losing their job 6
7 Changing your job 7
8 Personal experience of theft, mugging, break-in
   or another crime 8
9 Verbal abuse due to your race or colour 9
10 Physical attack due to your race or colour 0
11 Discrimination at work or anywhere else due
   to your race or colour X
12 Divorce, separation or break-up of an intimate
   relationship .... Y

(57)

13 Problems with your existing partner 1
14 Pregnancy 2
15 Problems with children 3
16 Problems with parents or close relatives 4
17 Moving home 5
18 Financial difficulties 6
19 Problems with neighbours 7

None of these 8
Don't know 9   (56-57)

Q86   SHOWCARD I (R)   Here is a list of health issues which can affect people's health. Can you tell me please which, if any, of these you feel have a bad effect on your health <u>at the moment</u>? Just read out the numbers of those you worry about.   MULTICODE OK

(58)

1.   The amount I smoke 1
2.   The kind of food I eat 2
3.   The quality of my housing 3
4.   Stress at home 4
5.   Living on my own 5
6.   The amount of alcohol I drink 6
7.   My weight 7
8.   Environmental pollution where I live 8
9.   Environmental pollution where I work 9
10. Environmental pollution in general 0
11. Stress at work X
12. My sexual behaviour .... Y

(59)

13. Road traffic in this area 1
14. Being unemployed 2
15. The amount of violent crime in this area 3
16. The amount of racism in this area 4
    Other (WRITE IN & CODE 5)

.... 5
None of these 6
Don't know 7   (58-59)

Q87   SHOWCARD J (R) **And which, if any, of these illnesses and health problems have you personally ever suffered from? Again, just call out the number.**

		(60)
1.	Severe arthritis/rheumatism	1
2.	Breathing difficulties eg bronchitis	2
3.	Cancer	3
4.	Depression/anxiety/nerves	4
5.	Alcoholism	5
6.	Stroke	6
7.	Degenerative diseases such as Multiple Sclerosis (MS), Parkinson's, osteoporosis	7
8.	HIV/AIDS	8
9.	Heart disease	9
10.	Back pain	0
11.	Diabetes	X
12.	STDs (sexually transmitted diseases)	Y
		(61)
13.	Anorexia nervosa	1
	Other (WRITE IN & CODE 2)	
	. . . .	2
	None of these	3
	Don't know	4

(60-61)

Q88   SHOWCARD K (R) **Looking at this card, which of these sentences best describes the amount of stress or pressure you experienced in the past 12 months?**

In the last 12 months, ...

	(62)
. . . . **I have been completely free of stress or pressure**	1
. . . . **I have experienced a small amount of stress or pressure**	2
. . . . **I have experienced a moderate amount of stress or pressure**	3
. . . . **I have experienced a large amount of stress or pressure**	4
Don't know	5

(62)

ASK WOMEN AGED 16-49

Q89   **(May I just check) Are you pregnant now?**

	(63)
Yes	1
No	2
Not sure	3

(63)

ASK ALL

Q90   **Can I just ask you how tall you are?** TAKE ESTIMATE IF NECESSARY

☐ feet   ☐☐ inches OR   ☐ m ☐☐ cms
(64)   (65) (66)   (67) (68) (69)   (64-69)

Q91   **And how much do you weigh at the moment?** TAKE ESTIMATE IF NECESSARY

☐☐ stone   ☐☐ pounds OR   ☐☐☐ kilogrammes
(70) (71)   (72) (73)   (74) (75) (76)   (70-76)

KNOWLEDGE

Q92 ASK ALL
SHOWCARD L (R) These are some terms relating to diet and eating. Which if any of these terms would you not feel confident explaining to someone else? Please call out all those that apply.

		(77)
1.	Cholesterol	1
2.	Fibre	2
3.	Energy	3
4.	Starchy foods	4
5.	Fats	5
6.	Polyunsaturated fat	6
7.	Saturated fat	7
8.	A balanced diet	8
9.	Carbohydrates	9
10.	Calories	0
11.	Vitamins	X
12.	E numbers or additives	Y
		(78)
	None of these	1
	Don't know	2

(77-78)

CARD ④ 10

Q93 SHOWCARD M (R)   Which, if any, of these can people do to reduce their chances of getting heart disease or a heart attack? MULTICODE OK

Q94 SHOWCARD M (R) AGAIN   Which, if any, of these can people do to reduce their chances of getting diabetes? MULTICODE OK

Q95 SHOWCARD M (R) AGAIN   Which, if any, of these can people do to reduce their chances of having a stroke? MULTICODE OK

Q96 SHOWCARD M (R) AGAIN   Which, if any, of these can people do to reduce their chances of getting osteoporosis? (That is bone loss) MULTICODE OK

		Q93 Heart disease (11)	Q94 Diabetes (13)	Q95 Stroke (15)	Q96 Osteo-porosis (17)
1.	Control bodyweight	1	1	1	1
2.	Reduce sugar intake	2	2	2	2
3.	Reduce fat intake	3	3	3	3
4.	Increase starch and fibre intake	4	4	4	4
5.	Eat a balanced diet	5	5	5	5
6.	Limit alcohol consumption	6	6	6	6
7.	Give up or cut down on smoking	7	7	7	7
8.	Eat plenty of fresh fruit and vegetables	8	8	8	8
9.	Reduce salt intake	9	9	9	9
10.	Take regular exercise	0	0	0	0
11.	Reduce stress	X	X	X	X
	None of these	Y	Y	Y	Y
		(12)	(14)	(16)	(18)
	Don't know	1	1	1	1

(11-18)

Q97　SHOWCARD N (R)　**Which of the foods on this card do you think are high . . .** (READ OUT EACH HEADING)?　**Just read out the numbers of the ones which apply.**　MULTICODE OK
ROTATE ORDER.　TICK START.

		Starch ☐ (19)	Fat ☐ (21)	Saturated fat ☐ (23)
1)	Red meat	1	1	1
2)	Chicken	2	2	2
3)	White fish (not fried)	3	3	3
4)	Pies, pasties, quiches	4	4	4
5)	Pasta and noodles	5	5	5
6)	Potatoes (not chips)	6	6	6
7)	Whole milk	7	7	7
8)	Cheese	8	8	8
9)	Soft margarine	9	9	9
10)	Fruit	0	0	0
11)	Butter	X	X	X
12)	Crisps	Y	Y	Y
		(20)	(22)	(24)
13)	Biscuits	1	1	1
	None of these	2	2	2
	Don't know	3	3	3　(19-24)

Q98　**How would you describe a healthy diet?**　PROBE:　**What would it contain?**　WRITE IN

```
.............................................................. (25)
                                                              1 2 3 4
                                                              5 6 7 8
                                                              9 0 X Y
.............................................................. (26)
                                                              1 2 3 4
                                                              5 6 7 8
                                                              9 0 X Y
.............................................................. (27)
                                                              1 2 3 4
                                                              5 6 7 8
..............................................................  9 0 X Y
```

Q99　SHOWCARD O (R)　**On this card we have grouped together some foods which are similar. Thinking about each group of foods as a whole, are there any groups of foods on this card which you think you personally eat too much of?**　IF YES:　**Which ones?**　MULTICODE OK

Q100　SHOWCARD O (R) AGAIN　**And which if any of these groups do you think you eat too little of?**　MULTICODE OK

	Q99 (28)	Q100 (29)
Bread/cereal/potatoes/rice/pasta and noodles	1	1
Fruit/vegetables	2	2
Milk and dairy (including yoghurt, cheese)	3	3
Meat and alternatives (poultry, fish, eggs, beans and lentils, cheese)	4	4
Fatty foods, cakes and sweets (including fatty meat, sausages, luncheon meat, crisps, biscuits, rich sauces/ gravies, cream, cream cheese, pastries, pies, cakes, doughnuts, chocolate, ice cream)	5	5
Fats (butter/margarine/low fat spread/vegetable oils/ mayonnaise/oily salad dressing)	6	6
Other (WRITE IN AND CODE '7')	7	7
None	8	8
Don't know	9	9　(28-29)

FOOD BUYING

Q101 **I would now like to ask you some questions about buying food. Do you do most of the food shopping for this household or does somebody else?** PROBE WHO. MULTICODE OK

	(30)	
Respondent	1	ASK Q102
Other household member		
- wife	2	
- girlfriend/partner	3	
- mother/mother-in-law	4	
- other female household member	5	
- husband	6	
- boyfriend/partner	7	
- father/father-in-law	8	
- other male household member	9	
Other (WRITE IN AND CODE '0')		
....	0	
Don't know	X	(30)

ASK Q102 IF CODE 1 AT Q101 - OTHERS GO TO Q108

Q102 SHOWCARD P (R) **Which one of the places on this list do you buy most of your food in?** (MULTICODE OK IF EQUAL)

	(31)	
Small local shops	1	
Local supermarkets	2	
Supermarkets in other towns or other parts of town	3	
Markets	4	
Food halls in department stores	5	ASK Q103
Farms and farm stalls	6	
Mobile shops	7	
Other	8	
Don't know	9	GO TO Q104 (31)

ASK ABOUT OUTLET MENTIONED AT Q102

Q103 **And why do you do most of your shopping in .... (OUTLET)?** MULTICODE OK

	(32)
Prices are affordable	1
Good range of healthy choices	2
Good quality food	3
Quick or convenient to get to	4
Foods are fresh	5
Wide range of foods available	6
Shop/outlet is clean	7
Sell things other than foods/can do all shopping in same place	8
My family or friends go there	9
I've always done my shopping there	0
Other (WRITE IN & CODE 'X')	
....	X
Don't know	Y (32)

Q104 **How do you usually travel to the place you do most of your food shopping?**

	(33)
Walk	1
Car	2 ASK Q105
Bus	3
Train/tube	4
Bicycle	5
Motorbike	6
Other (WRITE IN & CODE 7)	
	7
Don't know	8 (33)

ASK IF CAR MENTIONED AT Q104
Q105 **Is that your own car or someone else's?**

	(34)
Own car/household's car (including company car)	1
Car belongs to someone outside household	2 (34)

ASK ALL FOOD SHOPPERS (CODE 1 AT Q101)
Q106 **When you go food shopping, what factors do you think affect the choice of foods you buy?** DO NOT PROMPT. CODE BELOW

	(35)
The cost of foods/my food budget	1
Not eating certain foods because advised not to by health professional/ eating certain foods because advised to/medically prescribed diet	2
What my spouse/partner will eat	3
What my child/children will eat	4
Trying to eat a healthy balanced diet	5
The kind of foods I like eating	6
Convenience	7
Whether my spouse/partner is with me	8
Whether my child/children are with me	9
Packaging/display	0
Food advertising	X
Programmes/news items about food in media (TV/radio/papers)	Y
	(36)
The kind of foods my friends buy	1
The kind of foods my relatives buy	2
Whether I'm hungry or not	3
Religious/cultural reasons	4
Vegetarian/vegan	5
Other (WRITE IN & CODE '6')	
	6
Don't know	7 (35-36)

Q107 SHOWCARD P (R)   **Which if any of these do you think limit the choice of food you buy?**

	(37)
Ability to store food	1
Limited cooking facilities	2
Don't know how to cook some foods	3
Ability to carry and transport foods	4
Food goes off before it's eaten	5
Difficult to get to shops with children	6
Difficult to get to shops because of age or disability	7
Other (WRITE IN & CODE 8)	
	8
None of these	9
Don't know	0 (37)

ASK ALL

Q108 SHOWCARD Q (R) **How strongly do you agree or disagree with the following statements?**
READ OUT. ROTATE ORDER. TICK START.

		Strongly agree	Tend to agree	Neither agree nor disagree	Tend to disagree	Strongly disagree	Don't know	

The shops that serve my local community :

☐ a) ... have a good supply of fresh fruit and vegetables ..... 1 ..... 2 ..... 3 ..... 4 ..... 5 .... <u>6</u> (38)

b) ... have good quality fresh fruit and vegetables .... 1 ..... 2 ..... 3 ..... 4 ..... 5 .... 6 (39)

c) ... do not sell dairy products that have a reduced fat content .... 1 ..... 2 ..... 3 ..... 4 ..... 5 .... 6 (40)

☐ d) ... only have pre-packaged frozen meats, not fresh meat ... 1 ..... 2 ..... 3 ..... 4 ..... 5 .... 6 (41)

e) ... generally have fresh baked bread .... 1 ..... 2 ..... 3 ..... 4 ..... 5 .... 6 (42)

f) ... have a good supply of pasta/noodles/rice etc .... 1 ..... 2 ..... 3 ..... 4 ..... 5 .... 6 (43)

g) ... are generally more expensive than elsewhere ..... 1 ..... 2 ..... 3 ..... 4 ..... 5 .... 6 (44)

☐ h) ... do not provide information on healthy eating .... 1 ..... 2 ..... 3 ..... 4 ..... 5 .... 6 (45)

BARRIERS TO EATING GROUPS OF FOODS

ASK ALL
Q109   SHOWCARD R (R) **Looking at this list, are there any types of food here which you never or rarely eat for any reason? Just call out the numbers.**

ASK ABOUT EACH FOOD MENTIONED
Q110   SHOWCARD S (R)   **Why do you not eat . . . (FOOD)?** MULTICODE OK

Q110

		Q109	Don't like the taste	Price	Incon-venient/ difficult to prepare	Can't buy it in shops	Bad for you	Makes you fat	Religious or cultural reasons/ vege-tarian/ vegan	Other	Don't know	
		(46)										(46-47)
1)	Red meat (apart from sausages and burgers)	1	1	2	3	4	5	6	7	8	9	(48)
	IF 'OTHER' CODED, WRITE IN											
2)	Chicken	2	1	2	3	4	5	6	7	8	9	(49)
	IF 'OTHER' CODED, WRITE IN											
3)	Fish (not fried)	3	1	2	3	4	5	6	7	8	9	(50)
	IF 'OTHER' CODED, WRITE IN											
4)	Pulses such as beans and lentils	4	1	2	3	4	5	6	7	8	9	(51)
	IF 'OTHER' CODED, WRITE IN											
5)	Pasta/noodles/rice/ potatoes apart from chips	5	1	2	3	4	5	6	7	8	9	(52)
	IF 'OTHER' CODED, WRITE IN											
6)	Bread or chapatis	6	1	2	3	4	5	6	7	8	9	(53)
	IF 'OTHER' CODED, WRITE IN											
7)	Vegetables and salads	7	1	2	3	4	5	6	7	8	9	(54)
	IF 'OTHER' CODED, WRITE IN											
8)	Fruit	8	1	2	3	4	5	6	7	8	9	(55)
	IF 'OTHER' CODED, WRITE IN											
9)	Skimmed/semi-skimmed milk	9	1	2	3	4	5	6	7	8	9	(56)
	IF 'OTHER' CODED, WRITE IN											
10)	Sunflower/polyunsaturated margarine	0	1	2	3	4	5	6	7	8	9	(57)
	IF 'OTHER' CODED, WRITE IN											
11)	Low-fat spreads	X	1	2	3	4	5	6	7	8	9	(58)
	IF 'OTHER' CODED, WRITE IN											
12)	Eggs	Y	1	2	3	4	5	6	7	8	9	(59)
	IF 'OTHER' CODED, WRITE IN											
		(47)										
13)	Cheese	1	1	2	3	4	5	6	7	8	9	(60)
	IF 'OTHER' CODED, WRITE IN											

None of these 2

Don't know 3

HEALTHY EATING/DIETARY CHANGE

Q111 SHOWCARD Q (R) AGAIN How strongly do you agree or disagree with the following statements?
READ OUT
ROTATE ORDER. TICK START.

		Strongly agree	Tend to agree	Neither agree nor disagree	Tend to disagree	Strongly dis-agree	Don't know	
☐	a)	Healthy eating is just another fashion	1	2	3	4	5	6	(61)
	b)	I mostly eat a healthy diet nowadays	1	2	3	4	5	6	(62)
	c)	It's not very easy to eat healthy foods if you eat out	1	2	3	4	5	6	(63)
	d)	Eating healthy food is expensive	1	2	3	4	5	6	(64)
	e)	Healthy foods are enjoyable	1	2	3	4	5	6	(65)
	f)	The tastiest foods are the ones that are bad for you	1	2	3	4	5	6	(66)
☐	g)	I don't really care what I eat	1	2	3	4	5	6	(67)
	h)	I get confused over what's supposed to be healthy and what isn't	1	2	3	4	5	6	(68)
	i)	Experts never agree about what foods are good for you	1	2	3	4	5	6	(69)

ASK THOSE WHO LIVE WITH SPOUSE/PARTNER

	j)	My partner always wants to eat the foods he/she is familiar with	1	2	3	4	5	6	(70)
	k)	My partner often persuades me to buy unhealthy foods	1	2	3	4	5	6	(71)

ASK PARENTS

☐	l)	Feeding my family what they like is more important than trying to eat healthy foods	1	2	3	4	5	6	(72)
	m)	My child/ren always want to eat the foods they're familiar with	1	2	3	4	5	6	(73)
	n)	My child/ren often persuade me to buy unhealthy foods	1	2	3	4	5	6	(74)

Q112 **Can you tell me what changes, if any, you personally could make to have a healthier diet?**
MULTICODE OK

(75)

Eat less:

- generally 1
- convenience foods/fast foods/takeaways 2
- fat 3
- red meat/fatty meat 4
- fried food 5
- sugar/sweets/chocolates/biscuits/cakes 6
- eggs 7

Drink less:

- alcohol 8
- whole milk 9
- fizzy drinks (eg coke) 0

Switched to:

- lower fat food X
- lean meats . . . . Y

(76)

- polyunsaturated/monounsaturated fats (Flora,
    sunflower oil, olive oil etc) 1
- low fat spreads 2
- skimmed/semi-skimmed milk 3

Eat more:

- high fibre food (eg granary/wholemeal bread,
    pulses, bran cereals) 4
- starchy food (rice, pasta, potatoes, bread, cereals) 5
- fruit/vegetables/salad 6
- fish 7
- lean meat 8

Change cooking methods (eg grilling instead of frying) 9
Join a Slimming Club/Class (eg Weight Watchers) 0
Go to see my doctor or a dietician X
Take vitamin/mineral tablets . . . . Y

(77)

Take other food supplements 1
Buy meal replacements/special prepared foods for people
on a diet (eg Slimfast) 2
Other (WRITE IN AND CODE 3)

. . . . 3

None, no changes necessary 4
Don't know 5   (75-77)

Q113 **In what ways, if any, have you changed your diet over the last three years?**
MULTICODE OK

(78)

Eat less:
- generally 1
- convenience foods/fast foods/takeaways 2
- fat 3
- red meat/fatty meat 4
- fried food 5
- sugar/sweets/chocolates/biscuits/cakes 6
- eggs 7

Drink less:
- alcohol 8
- whole milk 9
- fizzy drinks (eg coke) 0

Switched to:
- lower fat food X
- lean meats .... Y

(79)

- polyunsaturated/monounsaturated fats (flora,
  sunflower oil, olive oil etc) 1
- low fat spreads 2
- skimmed/semi-skimmed milk 3

Eat more:
- high fibre food (eg granary/wholemeal bread,
  pulses, bran cereals) 4
- starchy food (rice, pasta, potatoes, bread, cereals) 5
- fruit/vegetables/salad 6
- fish 7
- lean meat 8

Change cooking methods (eg grilling instead of frying) 9
Join a Slimming Club/Class (eg Weight Watchers) 0
Go to see my doctor or a dietician X
Take vitamin/mineral tablets .... Y

(80)

Take other food supplements 1
Buy meal replacements/special prepared foods for people
on a diet (eg Slimfast) 2
Other (WRITE IN AND CODE 3)

.... 3

None (no changes) .... 4 ⎫ GO TO Q116
Don't know .... 5 ⎭

(78-80)
CARD ⑤   10

ASK ALL EXCEPT NONE/DON'T KNOW AT Q113
Q114 SHOWCARD T (R) **For what reasons have you made an effort to eat a healthier diet?**

(11)

Hospital admission/attendance 1
Illness or generally feeling unwell 2
Ill health in partner/close friend/relative 3
Health check 4
To lose weight 5
Ethical or religious reasons 6
To improve my health generally 7
To feel better mentally 8
Travel abroad 9
Advice from health professionals 0
More money available to spend on food X
Other (WRITE IN & CODE Y)

.... Y

(12)

No particular reason 1
Don't know 2   (11-12)

Q115 **What benefits, if any, do you think you have gained from making these changes to your diet?**

	(13)
Feel a lot healthier generally	1
Have lost weight	2
Blood cholesterol down	3
Blood pressure down	4
Less risk of heart disease	5
Less risk of bowel cancer	6
Less risk of other serious illnesses/disease	7
Fitter/more mobile	8
Easier to control my weight	9
Feel a sense of achievement/feel better mentally	0
My physical appearance has improved	X
Other (WRITE IN AND CODE Y)	

.... Y	
	(14)
None/No benefits	1
Don't know	2

(13-14)

ASK Q116 OF THOSE WHO SAID "NONE" AT Q113 OTHERS GO TO Q117

Q116 SHOWCARD U (R) **Looking at this card, which of these best describes your reasons for not having made an effort to eat a healthy diet over the last three years? Just read out the letters.**

		(15)
A.	Already eating a healthy diet	1
B.	Not interested/cannot be bothered/don't believe it's important for me	2
C.	None of the experts seem to agree so why should I change	3
D.	I don't know enough about which foods are good for you	4
E.	It's too expensive	5
F.	Pressure/resistance to change from spouse/partner	6
G.	Pressure/resistance to change from children	7
H.	I don't really believe the food you eat affects your health	8
I.	Not enough time to cook/prepare/buy healthy foods	9
J.	I don't need to worry about the food I eat at my age	0
K.	I like the taste of the food that I already eat	X
L.	I take plenty of exercise therefore I can eat what I like	Y
		(16)
M.	Now I have less money to spend on food	1
N.	I wouldn't enjoy eating healthier foods	2
O.	Travel/moving around	3
P.	Difficult to get access to cooking facilities	4
Q.	Family upset/disruption	5
R.	Other responsibilities mean I don't have time to cook for myself	6
	Other (WRITE IN AND CODE 7)	

.... 7	
Don't know	8

(15-16)

ASK ALL

Q117 **If you wanted to change your diet in order to control your weight, what changes would you make, if any? What others?**

Eat less: (17)

- generally 1
- convenience foods/fast foods/takeaways 2
- fat 3
- red meat/fatty meat 4
- fried food 5
- sugar/sweets/chocolates/biscuits/cakes 6
- eggs 7

Drink less:

- alcohol 8
- whole milk 9
- fizzy drinks (eg coke) 0

Switched to:

- lower fat food X
- lean meats . . . . Y
  (18)
- polyunsaturated/monounsaturated fats (flora, sunflower oil, olive oil etc) 1
- low fat spreads 2
- skimmed/semi-skimmed milk 3

Eat more:

- high fibre food (eg granary/wholemeal bread, pulses, bran cereals) 4
- starchy food (rice, pasta, potatoes, bread, cereals) 5
- fruit/vegetables/salad 6
- fish 7
- lean meat 8

Change cooking methods (eg grilling instead of frying) 9
Join a Slimming Club/Class (eg Weight Watchers) 0
Go to see my doctor or a dietician X
Take vitamin/mineral tablets . . . . Y
  (19)
Take other food supplements 1
Buy meal replacements/special prepared foods for people on a diet (eg Slimfast) 2

Other (WRITE IN AND CODE 3)

. . . . 3

None (no changes necessary) 4
Don't know 5   (17-19)

COOKING FACILITIES AND SKILLS

ASK ALL
Q118 **Last week, how many main meals did you eat at home? (I mean, your main meal of the day).**

(20)

□

Away from home last week . . . . Y GO TO Q122   (20)

(ASK IF Y NOT CODED AT Q118)
Q119 **How many of your main meals last week were meals bought ready-prepared, for example from a supermarket?**

(21)

□

(21)

Q120 **And how many were take-aways?**

(22)

□

(22)

Q121 **And how many were eaten out, for example in a restaurant?**

(23)

□

(23)

ASK ALL
Q122 SHOWCARD V (R) **How often do you cook a meal? (Any meal, not just main meals)**

(24)
Everyday 1
Most days (5 or 6 days a week) 2
Some days (3 or 4 days a week) 3   ASK Q123
One or two days a week 4
Less than once a week 5
Only for special occasions/dinner parties 6
Never 7
Don't know 8   GO TO Q124   (24)

ASK IF CODES 1-6 AT Q122
Q123 SHOWCARD W (R) **How easy or difficult is it normally for you to use cooking facilities when you want to?**

(25)
Very easy 1
Fairly easy 2
Fairly difficult 3
Very difficult 4
Don't know 5   (25)

ASK ALL
Q124 SHOWCARD X (R) **Which if any of these does your household use when cooking or preparing meals?**

(26)
a) A separate kitchen just for your own household's use 1
b) A separate kitchen which you have to
    share with other households 2
c) Cooking facilities just for your household's
    use but not in a separate room 3

Something else 4
Don't know 5   (26)

Q125 SHOWCARD Y (R) Which room do you normally eat your meals in?

		(27)
a)	Living room, at a table	1
b)	Living room, in front of the TV	2
c)	Dining room, at a table	3
d)	Kitchen	4
	It depends	6
	Never eat at home	7

Other (WRITE IN & CODE 5)

. . . . 5 _____ (27)

Q126 SHOWCARD Z (R)   And which if any of these does your household have the use of?
MULTICODE OK

	(28)
Cooker with four rings	1
Cooker with two rings	2
Oven	3
Grill	4
Electric frying-pan	5
Microwave oven	6
Combined fridge-freezer	7
Refrigerator	8
Separate freezer	9
Other (WRITE IN AND CODE 0)	

. . . . 0

None of these	X
Don't know	Y

_____ (28)

Q127 SHOWCARD AA (R) And which if any of these smaller pieces of kitchen equipment does your
household have the use of? MULTICODE OK

	(29)
Non-stick pans or woks	1
Steamer	2
Food processor	3
Liquidiser	4
Chip pan or deep fat fryer	5
Slow cooker	6
Pressure cooker	7
None of these	8
Don't know	9

_____ (29)

Q128 SHOWCARD BB (R) How confident do you feel about being able to cook from basic ingredients
as opposed to using convenience foods or cook-chill dishes?

	(30)
Very confident	1
Fairly confident	2
Not very confident	3
Not at all confident	4
Never use convenience foods or cook-chill dishes	5
Don't cook	6
Don't know	7

_____ (30)

Q129 SHOWCARD CC (R) **Which, if any of these cooking techniques do you feel confident about using? MULTICODE OK**

		(31)
1.	Boiling	1
2.	Steaming	2
3.	Shallow frying	3
4.	Deep frying	4
5.	Grilling	5
6.	Poaching	6
7.	Oven-baking or roasting	7
8.	Stewing/braising/casseroling	8
9.	Microwaving	9
10.	Stir frying	0
	None of these	X
	Don't know	Y (31)

Q130 SHOWCARD DD (R) **Which, if any of these foods do you feel confident about cooking? MULTICODE OK**

		(32)
1.	Red meat	1
2.	Chicken	2
3.	White fish (such as cod, haddock, plaice)	3
4.	Oily fish (such as herring, mackerel, salmon)	4
5.	Pulses such as beans and lentils	5
6.	Pasta	6
7.	Rice (not rice pudding)	7
8.	Potatoes (not chips)	8
9.	Fresh green vegetables (eg cabbage, broccoli, spinach)	9
10.	Root vegetables (eg carrots, parsnips, swede)	0
	None of these	X
	Don't know	Y (32)

Q131 SHOWCARD EE (R) **How useful would you find more information on . . . ?** READ OUT ROTATE ORDER. TICK START.

	Very useful	Fairly useful	Not very useful	Not at all useful	Don't know	
☐ How to prepare vegetables and fruit	1	2	3	4	5	(33)
How to prepare meat and poultry	1	2	3	4	5	(34)
How to prepare fish	1	2	3	4	5	(35)
☐ Food hygiene	1	2	3	4	5	(36)
How to store perishable food safely	1	2	3	4	5	(37)
Safe use of the microwave to re-heat foods	1	2	3	4	5	(38)
☐ Microwave cookery generally	1	2	3	4	5	(39)

Q132 SHOWCARD FF (R) **How important do you think it is to teach children how to cook? I'd like you to think first of all just about boys.**

Q133 SHOWCARD FF (R) AGAIN **And how important do you think it is to teach girls to cook?**

	Q132 (40)	Q133 (41)
Very important	1	1
Fairly important	2	2
Not very important	3	3
Not at all important	4	4
Don't know	5	5 (40-41)

Q134   SHOWCARD GG (R)   When you first started learning to cook, which if any of these did you learn from? MULTICODE OK

Q135   SHOWCARD GG (R) AGAIN   And later on, which if any of these were useful to you in learning more about cooking? MULTICODE

	Q134 (42)	Q135 (44)
Mother	1	1
Father	2	2
Grandmother	3	3
Wife/husband/partner	4	4
Other relatives	5	5
Friends	6	6
Childminder	7	7
Cookery classes at school	8	8
Other cookery classes or courses (apart from school)	9	9
Cookery books	0	0
Cookery programmes on TV	X	X
Specialist cookery/food magazines	Y	Y
	(43)	(45)
Articles in magazines/newspapers	1	1
Booklets/leaflets from supermarkets	2	2
Booklets/leaflets from food producers	3	3
Health centre/doctor	4	4
None of these	5	5
Don't know	6	6
Haven't learnt to cook	7	GO TO Q136 (42-45)

Q136   Would you like to learn more about cooking?

	(46)		
Yes	1	GO TO Q138	
No	2	ASK Q137	
Don't know	3	GO TO Q138	(46)

ASK IF NO AT Q136

Q137   Why do you not want to learn more about cooking? MULTICODE OK

	(47)	
I know enough already	1	
Don't have time to cook	2	
Prefer to eat out/get takeaways/cook-chill foods	3	
Not interested in cooking	4	
Other (WRITE IN & CODE '5')		
....	5	
Don't know	6	(47)

ASK ALL

Q138   SHOWCARD HH (R)   If you wanted to find out more about cooking methods, which of these methods would you prefer to use? MULTICODE OK

	(48)	
Cookery programmes on TV	1	
Specialist cookery/food magazines	2	
Cookery books	3	
Cookery classes/courses	4	
Videos on Cookery Skills	5	
Ask a member of the family/friend	6	
Booklets/leaflets from supermarkets	7	
Articles in general interest newspapers/ magazines	8	
Booklets/leaflets from food producers	9	
Other (WRITE IN & CODE '0')		
....	0	
None of these	X	
Don't know	Y	
	(49)	
Wouldn't want find out more about healthier cooking methods	1	(48-49

FAMILY MEALS

ASK THOSE WHO DO NOT LIVE ALONE (THOSE LIVING ALONE GO TO Q143)
Q139   **Do you ever have a meal or snack at home with all or most of the other people in your household?**

		(50)		
Yes	....	1	ASK Q140	
No	....	2		
Don't know	....	3	GO TO Q143	(50)

ASK IF YES
Q140   SHOWCARD II (R) **About how often would you say you do this?**

		(51)	
Two or three times a day	....	1	
Once a day	....	2	
Every 2-3 days	....	3	
Every 4-5 days	....	4	
Once a week	....	5	
Less than once a week	....	6	
Don't know	....	7	(51)

Q141   SHOWCARD JJ (R)   **Which one of these statements best describes mealtimes with other members of your household?** SINGLE CODE ONLY

		(52)	
I usually enjoy mealtimes	....	1	
Sometimes I enjoy mealtimes sometimes not	......	2	
Mealtimes are not usually enjoyable	....	3	
Mealtimes are too rushed to notice whether they're enjoyable or not	....	4	
None of these	....	5	
Don't know	....	6	(52)

Q142   **Which meals or snacks, if any, do all members of your household eat together?** READ OUT IF NECESSARY MULTICODE OK

		(53)	
Sunday lunch	....	1	
Evening meals (on normal days)	....	2	
Breakfast	....	3	
Midday meals	....	4	
Sunday evening meal	....	5	
Other (WRITE IN & CODE '6')			
....		6	
None	....	7	
Don't know	....	8	(53)

MEALS AT WORK

ASK THOSE WHO WORK & ARE NOT SELF-EMPLOYED (CODES 1-2 AT Q5); OTHERS GO TO Q
Q143 **When you are at work, where do you usually obtain lunch? MULTICODE OK**

(54)

Workplace canteen or cafeteria 1
Pub 2
Cafe/takeaway/sandwich bar 3
Restaurant 4
Shop 5
Vending machine on-site 6
Vending machine off-site 7
Lunch supplied at meetings .... 8 } ASK Q144
Bring packed lunch from home 9
Often miss lunch/never have lunch 0
Don't have lunch at work (eg work evening/night shifts) .... X } GO TO Q145
Go home for lunch .... Y

(55)

Other (WRITE IN & CODE '1')

.... 1
Don't know 2 (54-55)

ASK IF CODES 1 TO 8 AT Q143 (OTHERS GO TO Q145)
Q144 **SHOWCARD KK (R) From this card, how would you describe the range of food available where you eat at lunchtime?**

(56)

Very good choice of healthy foods 1
Quite good choice of healthy foods 2
Satisfactory good choice of healthy foods 3
Quite poor choice of healthy foods 4
Very poor choice of healthy foods 5
Don't know 6 (56)

ASK THOSE WHO WORK & ARE NOT SELF-EMPLOYED
Q145 **Is the meal you eat at lunchtime on workdays ever your main meal of the day?**

(57)

Yes .... 1 ASK Q146
No 2
Don't know .... 3 } GO TO Q147 (57)

ASK IF YES AT Q145
Q146 **Thinking just about last week, how many times was your lunch time meal on workdays your main meal of the day? IF NONE ENTER '0'**

(58)

☐

(58)

CHOLESTEROL

ASK ALL
Q147   SHOWCARD LL (R) **How well informed do you feel about cholesterol?**

                                                                    (59)
              Very well informed 1
              Fairly well informed 2
              Not very well informed 3
              Not at all informed 4
              Don't know 5   (59)

Q148   **What, if any, are the health risks of having higher than average levels of cholesterol in your blood?** DO NOT PROMPT MULTICODE OK

                                                                    (60)
       Increased risk of:

              Overweight/obesity 1
              High blood pressure 2
              Coronary heart disease 3
              Heart attack 4
              Stroke 5
              Gallstones 6
              Other (WRITE IN & CODE '7')

              7

       No health risks 8
       Don't know 9   (60)

Q149   SHOWCARD FF (R) AGAIN   **As far as you are aware, how important is each of the following in increasing your risk of getting coronary heart disease?**
       READ OUT. ALTERNATE ORDER. TICK START

	Very important	Fairly important	Not very important	Not at all important	Don't know	
☐ **Cholesterol**	1	2	3	4	5	(61)
Lack of exercise	1	2	3	4	5	(62)
Diet	1	2	3	4	5	(63)
☐ **Smoking**	1	2	3	4	5	(64)

Q150   SHOWCARD MM (R)   **Which if any of these statements describe cholesterol? Tell me all those you think are true.**

                                                                    (65)
       1   High blood cholesterol can be reduced by eating
              a diet low in saturated fat 1
       2   People only get raised cholesterol levels if it
              runs in their family 2
       3   Low cholesterol causes cancer 3
       4   Cholesterol comes only from the foods you eat 4
       5   One type of cholesterol in the blood is called
              serum cholesterol 5
       6   Only people with high blood pressure have high
              cholesterol 6
       7   High blood cholesterol can only be reduced by
              taking medication (drugs) 7

       None of these 8
       Don't know 9   (65)

Q151 **Have you ever had your blood cholesterol measured as far as you know?**

		(66)	
Yes	....	1	ASK Q152
No	....	2	GO TO
Don't know	....	3	Q161	(66)

ASK IF YES

Q152 **When was it (your first test, if you have had more than one)?**

		(67)
In last 3 months	....	1
In last 4-6 months	....	2
In last 7-12 months	....	3
Between 1 and 2 years ago	....	4
Over 2 years ago	....	5
Can't remember	....	6	(67)

Q153 **(On the first occasion you had your blood cholesterol measured), who if anyone was this suggested by?**

		(68)	
Family doctor/GP	....	1	
Chemist/pharmacist	....	2	
Practice nurse	....	3	GO TO Q155
Hospital staff	....	4	
Work doctor or nurse	....	5	
Family member or friend	....	6	
Just decided for myself	....	7	ASK Q154
Other (WRITE IN & CODE '8')			
....		8	GO TO Q155
Don't remember	....	9		(68)

ASK IF CODE 7 AT Q153

Q154 **What made you decide to have a cholesterol test?**

		(69)
Just interested	....	1
Though I might be at risk of heart disease/ heart attack	....	2
Family history of heart disease	....	3
Other family members have high cholesterol	....	4
Other (WRITE IN & CODE '5')		
....		5
Don't know	....	6	(69)

ASK ALL WHO HAVE HAD TEST

Q155 **And where did you get that test done?**

		(70)
At surgery/health centre	....	1
At hospital	....	2
At chemist's/pharmacist's	....	3
Through work	....	4
Other (WRITE IN & CODE '5')		
....		5
Can't remember	....	6	(70)

Q156 **What was the result of the test (your last one if you have had more than one)?**
READ OUT

			(71)
....	**Very high levels of cholesterol**	....	1
....	**High levels of cholesterol**	....	2
....	**Normal levels of cholesterol**	....	3
or .	**Lower than average levels of cholesterol**	....	4
Don't know		....	5	(71)

Q157 **Did you have any other tests done at the same time as your cholesterol test?** IF YES: **What other tests did you have done?**

(72)
Yes:
Blood pressure 1
Weight 2
Urine test 3
Body fat measure 4
Fitness/exercise test 5
Electrocardiogram 6
Other (WRITE IN & CODE '7')

.... 7

No other tests 8
Don't know/can't remember 9   (72)

Q158 **Were you asked for any other information about yourself at the same time?** IF YES; **What was that?**

(73)
No other information 1
Family medical history/family history
of heart disease 2
Dietary habits 3
Smoking habits/cigarette consumption 4
Drinking habits/alcohol consumption 5
Exercise habits 6
Other (WRITE IN & CODE '7') ....

.... 7
Don't know 8   (73)

Q159 **What advice, if any, did you get when you had your cholesterol test?**

(74)
Eat less fat 1
Eat less saturated fat 2
Change my diet 3
Gave me a diet sheet 4
Told me to eat less 5
Take more exercise 6
Smoke less/give up 7
Drink less alcohol 8
Relax, learn to reduce stress 9
Referred to hospital/specialist 0
Recommended to see GP X
Put on cholesterol-reducing drugs .... Y
(75)
Asked to come back for another test,
or referred elsewhere for another test 1

Other type of follow-up (WRITE IN & CODE '2') ......

.... 2

Other (WRITE IN AND CODE '3') ....

.... 3

No advice given 4

Can't remember 5   NOW GO TO Q163   (74-75)

ASK ALL EXCEPT 'NO ADVICE'/'CAN'T REMEMBER' AT Q159
Q160a How helpful did you find the advice you were given? Was it . . . READ OUT. ALTERNATE ORDER. TICK START

		(76)
☐	Very helpful	1
	Fairly helpful	2
	Not very helpful	3
☐	Not at all helpful	4
	Don't know	5	(76)

Q160b And did you follow any or all of the advice you were given, or not?

(77)
Yes, all 1
Yes, some 2
No, none 3
Can't remember 4   *NOW GO TO Q163*   (77)

ASK IF NOT HAD CHOLESTEROL TEST AT Q151
Q161 If you wanted a cholesterol test, where would you go or who would you talk to?

(78)
Surgery/health centre 1
Own GP/family doctor 2
Practice nurse 3
Get pharmacist/chemist to do test 4
Buy home testing kit from pharmacy/chemist 5
Other (WRITE IN AND CODE '6') . . . .

. . . . 6   (78)

Don't know 7

Q162 Why have you never had a cholesterol test? DO NOT PROMPT

(79)
Never been recommended to 1
Frightened/nervous of tests 2
Frightened/nervous of results 3
Don't want to do anything about my cholesterol level 4
Not worried about my cholesterol level/doesn't concern me 5
There's nothing I can do about it 6
Never thought about it 7
Don't want to bother doctor 8
Don't know who to talk to 9
Expensive 0
Too busy/never got round to it X
I'm not overweight . . . . Y
(80)
I eat a healthy diet 1
Heart disease doesn't run in my family 2
Other (WRITE IN AND CODE '3') . . . .

. . . . 3
Don't know 4   (79-80)

FAT/FIBRE CONSUMPTION

Q163　**Now I'd like to ask you some questions about how much you personally eat of certain types of food.**

　　a)　**First of all, about how many pieces of bread or rolls (or chapattis) do you eat on a usual day?**

　　b)　**Are they usually white, brown or wholemeal?**

　　　　INTERVIEWER: CODE AMOUNT EATEN AGAINST TYPE USUALLY EATEN
　　　　　　　　　　(SINGLE CODE ONLY)

	Less than 1 a day	1-2 a day	3-4 a day	5 or more a day	
White bread	1	2	3	4	(11)
Brown or granary bread	1	2	3	4	(12)
Wholemeal bread	1	2	3	4	(13)
Never eat bread/chapattis	1	2	3	4	(14)

Q164　a)　**About how many times a week do you have a bowl of breakfast cereal or porridge?**

　　b)　SHOWCARD OO (R)　**What kind do you have most often?**

　　　　INTERVIEWER: CODE NO OF TIMES AGAINST CEREAL EATEN MOST OFTEN
　　　　　　　　　　(SINGLE CODE ONLY)

	Less than 1 a week	1-2 a week	3-5 a week	6 or more a week	
Sugar types: Frosties, Coco Pops, Ricicles, Sugar Puffs etc	1	2	3	4	(15)
Rice/Corn type: Cornflakes, Rice Krispies, Special K etc	1	2	3	4	(16)
Porridge or Ready Brek etc	1	2	3	4	(17)
Wheat type: Shredded Wheat, Weetabix, Puffed Wheat, Fruit'n'Fibre, Nutri-grain, Oat Krunchies, Start etc	1	2	3	4	(18)
Muesli type: Alpen, Jordans etc	1	2	3	4	(19)
Bran type: All-bran, Bran Flakes, Sultana Bran, Team etc	1	2	3	4	(20)
Never eat cereal	X				

The questions on Fat and Fibre Consumption are derived from the DINE questionnaire (Dietary Instrument for Nutritional Education) designed by Liane Roe, ICRF General Practice Research Group, to whom we are indebted for permission to use them.

Q165 **About how many times a week do you eat the following foods?**
READ OUT EACH TYPE OF FOOD. (IF NONE/NEVER, CODE "LESS THAN 1")
NB: OTHER VEGETABLES' INCLUDES SALADS

	Less than 1 a week	1-2 a week	3-5 a week	6 or more a week	
Rice, spaghetti or noodles	1	2	3	4	(21)
Potatoes	1	2	3	4	(22)
Peas	1	2	3	4	(23)
Baked beans, dried beans or lentils	1	2	3	4	(24)
Other vegetables (any type)	1	2	3	4	(25)
Fruit (fresh, frozen or canned)	1	2	3	4	(26)

Q166 **About how many times a week do you eat a serving of the following foods?**
READ OUT EACH TYPE OF FOOD. (IF NONE/NEVER, CODE "LESS THAN 1")

	Less than 1 a week	1-2 a week	3-5 a week	6 or more a week	
Beefburgers or sausages	1	2	3	4	(27)
Beef, pork or lamb	1	2	3	4	(28)
Bacon, meat pies, processed meat	1	2	3	4	(29)
Chicken or turkey	1	2	3	4	(30)
Fish (NOT fried)	1	2	3	4	(31)

Q167 **About how many times a week do you eat a serving of the following foods?**
READ OUT EACH TYPE OF FOOD (IF NONE/NEVER, CODE "LESS THAN 1")

	Less than 1 a week	1-2 a week	3-5 a week	6 or more a week	
Cheese (any except cottage)	1	2	3	4	(32)
Any fried food; fried fish, chips cooked breakfast, samosas	1	2	3	4	(33)
Cakes pies, puddings, pastries	1	2	3	4	(34)
Biscuits, chocolate or crisps	1	2	3	4	(35)

Q168 a) **About how much milk do you yourself use in a day, for drinking or in cereal, tea, or coffee?**

b) **What kind of milk do you usually use?**

INTERVIEWER: CODE AMOUNT USED AGAINST TYPE USUALLY USED
(SINGLE CODE ONLY)

	Less than 1/4 pint	About a 1/4 pint	About a 1/2 pint	1 pint or more	
Full cream (silver top) or Channel Islands (gold top)	1	2	3	4	(36)
Semi-skimmed (red top)	1	2	3	4	(37)
Skimmed (blue top)	1	2	3	4	
Never drink/use milk	X				(38)

Q169 SHOWCARD PP (R) **What sort of fat do you use on bread and vegetables?** SINGLE CODE ONLY

Q170 SHOWCARD PP (R) AGAIN **And what sort of fat do you use for frying?** SINGLE CODE ONLY

Q171 SHOWCARD PP (R) AGAIN **And what sort of fat do you use for baking or cooking?** SINGLE CODE ONLY

		Q170 (39)	Q171 (40)	Q172 (41)
1)	Butter, ghee, dripping, lard, or solid cooking fat (White Cap, Cookeen)	1	1	1
2)	Hard margarine (Stork, Krona, Echo) Soft margarine (Stork Special Blend, Summer County, Mello) Solid sunflower oil (White Flora) Dairy blends (Clover, Golden Crown, Golden Crown Light, I Can't Believe It's Not Butter, Willow, Meadow Cup)	2	2	2
3)	Sunflower margarine (Flora, Vitalite, Vitalite Light, Blue Band Sunflower, supermarket brands) Olive margarine (Olivio, Olive Gold) Soya margarine	3	3	3
4)	Low fat spreads (St Ivel Gold, Outline, Flora Extra Light) Low fat dairy spreads (Delight, Clover Extra Light)	4	4	4
5)	Pure vegetable oil (eg sunflower, soya, corn, peanut, olive, rapeseed)	5	5	5
	None	6	6	6 (39-41)

Q172 a) **About how many pats or rounded teaspoons of margarine or butter do you usually use in a day, for example on bread, sandwiches, toast, potatoes, or vegetables?** WRITE IN

b) **And how many pats or rounded teaspoons of low fat spread?** WRITE IN

a) Butter or margarine ☐☐ pats/teaspoons (IF NONE, ENTER '00') (42-43)

b) Low fat spread ☐☐ pats/teaspoons (IF NONE, ENTER '00') (44-45)

SMOKING

Q173 **I would now like to ask you a few questions about smoking. Have you ever smoked a cigarette, a cigar or a pipe?**

(46)

Yes .... 1　ASK Q174
No .... 2　GO TO Q195　　　(46)

ASK ALL WHO EVER SMOKED. OTHERS GO TO Q195
Q174 **Do you smoke cigarettes at all nowadays?**

(47)

Yes .... 1　GO TO Q180
No .... 2　ASK Q175　　　(47)

ASK ALL WHO ARE NOT CURRENT CIGARETTE SMOKERS. OTHERS GO TO Q190
Q175 **How old were you when you first tried smoking?**

☐☐ years
(48) (49)　　　　　　　　　　　　　　　　　(48-49)

Q176 **Have you ever smoked cigarettes regularly?**

(50)

Yes .... 1　ASK Q177
No .... 2　GO TO Q190　　　(50)

Q177 **And how old were you when you started to smoke cigarettes regularly?**

☐☐ years
(51) (52)　　　　　　　　　　　　　　　　　(51-52)

Q178 **About how many cigarettes did you smoke in a day when you smoked them regularly?**

☐☐☐ cigarettes a day
(53) (54) (55)　　　　　　　　　　　　　　(53-55)

NB. IF 'ROLL YOUR OWN' GIVE AMOUNT OF TOBACCO

☐☐ GRAMMES
(56) (57)　　　　　　　　　　　　　　　　　(56-57)

Q179 **How long ago did you stop smoking cigarettes regularly?** IF LESS THAN 1 YEAR, GIVE ANSWER IN MONTHS

☐☐ years OR ☐☐ months
(58) (59)　　　　(60) (61)　　　　　　　　(58-61)

NOW GO TO Q 190

ASK CURRENT SMOKERS ONLY (YES AT Q174). OTHERS GO TO Q190

Q180   **How old were you when you first tried smoking?**

□□ years
(62) (63)   (62-63)

Q181   **Do you smoke cigarettes regularly nowadays?**

(64)
Yes 1   ASK Q182
No 2   GO TO Q185   (64)

Q182   **And how old were you when you started to smoke cigarettes regularly?**

□□ years
(65) (66)   (65-66)

Q183   **About how many cigarettes a day do you usually smoke on weekdays?**

□□□ cigarettes
(67) (68) (69)   (67-69)

NB. IF "ROLL YOUR OWN" GIVE AMOUNT OF TOBACCO

□□ GRAMMES
(70) (71)   (70-71)

Q184   **About how many cigarettes a day do you usually smoke at weekends?**

□□□ cigarettes
(72) (73) (74)   (72-74)

NB. IF "ROLL YOUR OWN" GIVE AMOUNT OF TOBACCO

□□ GRAMMES
(75) (76)   (75-76)

Q185   **Did you smoke any cigarettes yesterday?**

(77)
Yes 1   ASK Q186
No 2   GO TO Q187   (77)

Q186   **How many cigarettes did you smoke yesterday?**

□□□ cigarettes
(78) (79) (80)   (78-80)

NB. IF "ROLL YOUR OWN" GIVE AMOUNT OF TOBACCO   CARD⑦   10

□□ GRAMMES
(11) (12)   (11-12)

Q187 Have you ever tried to give up smoking?

Yes 1   ASK Q188

No 2   GO TO Q190   (13)

ASK IF YES AT Q187

Q188 And have you ever succeeded in giving up smoking for at least 12 months?

(14)

Yes 1   ASK Q189

No 2   GO TO Q190   (14)

ASK IF YES AT Q188

Q189 How long ago did you start smoking again? (the last time, if you have done this more than once)?
IF LESS THAN 1 YEAR, GIVE ANSWER IN MONTHS

□□ years   □□ months
(15) (16)   (17) (18)

Can't remember . . . . Y   (15-18)

ASK THOSE WHO HAVE EVER SMOKED AT Q173

Q190 Do you smoke at least one cigar of any kind per month nowadays?

(19)

Yes 1   ASK Q191

No 2   GO TO Q192   (19)

ASK IF YES AT Q190

Q191 About how many cigars do you usually smoke in a week?

□□
(20) (21)

Don't know . . . . Y   (20-21)

ASK IF NO AT Q190

Q192 Have you ever regularly smoked at least one cigar of any kind per month?

(22)

Yes 1

No 2   (22)

ASK ALL MEN WHO HAVE EVER SMOKED AT Q173

Q193 Do you smoke a pipe at all nowadays?

(23)

Yes 1   GO TO Q195

No 2   ASK Q194   (23)

ASK IF NO AT Q193

Q194 Have you ever smoked a pipe regularly?

(24)

Yes 1

No 2   (24)

INTERVIEWER: FIRST RECORD BELOW RESPONDENT'S SMOKING STATUS. THEN FOR THOSE WHO DO NOT LIVE ALONE, REFER BACK TO PERSON NUMBERS ON P1. TO REMIND YOURSELF WHICH NUMBER REFERS TO WHICH HOUSEHOLD MEMBER. IN THE QUESTIONS WHICH FOLLOW, THE PERSON NUMBER MUST REFER TO THE SAME ACTUAL PERSON AS BEFORE.

ASK FOR EACH OTHER HOUSEHOLD MEMBER
Q195 Does he/she smoke, as far as you know? IF YES, CODE AS CURRENT SMOKER

ASK FOR EACH ONE WHO DOES NOT SMOKE
Q196 Has he/she ever smoked? IF YES, CODE AS EX-SMOKER; IF NO, AS NEVER SMOKED

	(Respondent)			Person Number		
	Person 1	2	3	4	5	6
	(25)	(26)	(27)	(28)	(29)	(30)
Current smoker	1	1	1	1	1	1
Ex-smoker	2	2	2	2	2	2
Never smoked	3	3	3	3	3	3
Don't know	4	4	4	4	4	4

IF NO SMOKERS IN HH, NOW GO TO Q201

ASK RESPONDENTS WHO SMOKE
Q197 Do you ever smoke when at home?

ASK ABOUT EACH OTHER HH MEMBER WHO SMOKES
Q198 Does he/she ever smoke when at home, as far as you know?

	Q197	Q198				
	Person 1	Person 2	Person 3	Person 4	Person 5	Person 6
Smokes at home	5	5	5	5	5	5
Doesn't smoke at home	6	6	6	6	6	6
Don't know	7	7	7	7	7	7 (25-30)

ASK RESPONDENTS WHO SMOKE
Q199 Where in the home do you normally smoke? MULTICODE OK

ASK ABOUT EACH OTHER HH MEMBER WHO SMOKES
Q200 Where in the home does he/she normally smoke? MULTICODE OK

	Q199			Q200		
	Person 1	Person 2	Person 3	Person 4	Person 5	Person 6
	(31)	(32)	(33)	(34)	(35)	(36)
Everywhere	1	1	1	1	1	1
Own room/bedroom	2	2	2	2	2	2
Living room	3	3	3	3	3	3
Kitchen	4	4	4	4	4	4
Toilet	5	5	5	5	5	5
Bathroom	6	6	6	6	6	6
Outdoors only	7	7	7	7	7	7
Other	8	8	8	8	8	8
Nowhere	9	9	9	9	9	9
Don't know	0	0	0	0	0	0 (31-36)

ASK ALL
Q201 Do you have any rules about whether people should smoke in your home or where they should smoke?

	(37)
Yes	1
No	2
Don't know	3 (37)

ASK ALL
Q202 SHOWCARD **Which of these best describes what happens when you have visitors in your home?**

(38)

All visitors are allowed to smoke in my home,
  if they wish .... 1 GO TO Q204
Some visitors are allowed to smoke in my home,
  others are not .... 2 ASK Q203
No visitors are allowed to smoke in my home .... 3 GO TO Q204
We never have visitors who might want to smoke .... 4 ⎱
We never have visitors .... 5 ⎰ GO TO
It depends 6   Q206
Don't know .... 7 ⎰

(38)

ASK IF CODE 2 AT Q202 (SOME VISITORS ALLOWED TO SMOKE)
Q203 **What sorts of visitors would be allowed to smoke in your home?** MULTICODE OK

(39)

Parents 1
Parents-in-law 2
Friends 3
Children 4
Children's friends 5
Other relatives 6
Other (WRITE IN AND CODE '7') 7

....

....

It depends 8
Don't know 9

(39)

ASK IF CODES 1, 2, 3 AT Q202
Q204 SHOWCARD QQ(R) **If you did not want visitors to smoke in your home how confident would you feel about asking them not to?**

(40)

Very confident .... 1 ⎱ GO TO Q206
Fairly confident .... 2 ⎰
Not very confident .... 3 ⎱ ASK Q205
Not at all confident .... 4 ⎰
Don't know 5   GO TO Q206

(40)

IF NOT VERY/NOT AT ALL CONFIDENT AT Q204
Q205 **Why would you not feel confident about asking visitors not to smoke in your home?**

(41)

Not up to me to decide who smokes here 1
Feel too embarrassed to ask 2
Don't want to lay down the law/be bossy 3
Don't want to make a fuss 4
Don't want to offend people 5
Don't want to be unfriendly/make people
  feel rejected 6
Other (WRITE IN & CODE '7')

.... 7
Don't know 8

(41)

ASK ALL SMOKERS (YES AT Q174). OTHERS GO TO Q208

Q206 SHOWCARD RR(R) **Which of these places, if any, did you smoke in, yesterday?**
MULTICODE OK

	(42)
At home	1
At work	2
At the pub	3
At a friend's/relative's home	4
Outdoors	5
In restaurants/canteens	6
In shops	7
Whilst travelling by car	8
On the train	9
On the bus	0
On the underground	X
In a taxi cab	Y

(43)

Other (WRITE IN AND CODE 1) . . . .

. . . .

. . . . 1

None of these places 2
Don't know 3   (42-43)

Q207 SHOWCARD SS(R) **Are there any places or situations on this card where you feel you shouldn't smoke? Which ones?**

	(44)
Doctors' surgeries/health centres	1
Hospital waiting areas	2
Restaurants/places where people are eating nearby	3
The homes of people who do not smoke	4
Near babies/young children	5
Near pregnant women	6
On public transport	7
Other public places	8
When with other people who are eating	9
Aeroplanes	0
Shops	X
Public toilets	Y

(45)

In the street	1
All places where there is a smoking ban	2
During pregnancy	3

Other (WRITE IN & CODE '4') . . . .

. . . . 4
None 5
Don't know 6   (44-45)

ASK ALL
Q208 SHOWCARD TT(R) **Do you ever visit any of these places?**

ASK FOR EACH PLACE
Q209 SHOWCARD UU(R) **From this card, how would you normally visit . . . (PLACE), when you do go there?** MULTICODE OK

Q209

	Q208 (46)	Alone	With spouse/ partner	With family	With friends	It depends	Don't know (46)
Restaurants	1	1	2	3	4	5	6 (47)
Cafe's/takeaways	2	1	2	3	4	5	6 (48)
Pubs	3	1	2	3	4	5	6 (49)
Cinemas	4	1	2	3	4	5	6 (50)
Friends' homes	5	1	2	3	4	5	6 (51)
None of these	6	GO TO Q215					

ASK FOR EACH TYPE OF PLACE VISITED AT Q208

Q210 SHOWCARD VV(R) **How much does the amount of cigarette smoke in restaurants affect your choice of which restaurants you go to?**

Q211 SHOWCARD VV(R) AGAIN **How much does the amount of cigarette smoke in cafe's and takeaways   affect your choice of which cafe's and takeaways you go to?**

Q212 SHOWCARD VV(R) AGAIN **How much does the amount of cigarette smoke in pubs affect your choice of which pubs you go to?**

Q213 SHOWCARD VV(R) AGAIN **How much does the amount of cigarette smoke in cinemas affect your choice of which cinemas you go to?**

Q214 SHOWCARD VV(R) AGAIN **How much does the amount of cigarette smoke in friends' homes affect your choice of which friends' homes you go to?**

	Q210 Rest-aurants (52)	Q211 Cafe's/ take-aways (53)	Q212 Pubs (54)	Q213 Cinemas (55)	Q214 Friends' homes (56)
A great deal	1	1	1	1	1
A fair amount	2	2	2	2	2
A little	3	3	3	3	3
Not at all	4	4	4	4	4
I/we would never go somewhere with a smoky atmosphere	5	5	5	5	5
None of my friends smoke					6
It depends	7	7	7	7	7
Don't know	8	8	8	8	8 (52-56)

ASK ALL

Q215 **About how much time would you say you spend in an average day in places where you are inhaling other people's cigarette smoke?** IF LESS THAN 1 HR, RECORD IN MINUTES

☐☐ hours
(57) (58)

☐☐ minutes
(59) (60)

None X
Don't know .... Y   (57-60)

ASK ALL SMOKERS (YES AT Q174)

Q216 SHOWCARD WW(R) **How much, if at all, would you say your smoking affects your health?**

	(61)	
A great deal	1	
A fair amount	2	ASK Q217
Just a little	3	
Not at all	4	
Don't know	5	GO TO Q218 (61)

ASK IF CODES 1-3 AT Q216

Q217 **In what ways would you say your smoking affects your health?** DO NOT PROMPT

	(62)
Breathlessness	1
Coughing	2
Wheezing	3
Get asthma/makes asthma worse	4
Prone to chest infections/bronchitis	5
Less fit than I used to be	6
Worry about serious illness	7
Likely to suffer from cancer	8
Likely to suffer from another serious illness (SPECIFY & CODE 9)	
....	9
General poor health	0
Other (WRITE IN AND CODE X	
....	X
Don't know	Y

(62)

ASK ALL

Q218 **SHOWCARD WW(R) AGAIN How much, if at all, would you say passive smoking affects people who are exposed to it?**

	(63)	
A great deal	1	
A fair amount	2	ASK Q219
Just a little	3	
Not at all	4	
It depends	5	GO TO Q220
Don't know	6	

(63)

ASK IF CODES 1-3 AT Q218

Q219 **In what ways would you say passive smoking affects people's health?**

	(64)
Breathlessness	1
Coughing	2
Wheezing	3
Get asthma/make asthma worse	4
Prone to chest infections/bronchitis	5
Less fit than he/she used to be	6
Worry about serious illness	7
Likely to suffer from cancer	8
Likely to suffer from another serious illness (SPECIFY & CODE 9)	
....	9
General poor health	0
Other (WRITE IN & CODE X)	
....	X
Don't know	Y

(64)

ASK ALL

Q220 **SHOWCARD WW(R) AGAIN How much, if at all, would you say passive smoking affects pregnant women?**

	(65)	
A great deal	1	
A fair amount	2	ASK Q221
Just a little	3	
Not at all	4	GO TO Q222
Don't know	5	

(65)

ASK IF CODES 1-3 AT Q220
Q221 In what ways would you say passive smoking affects pregnant women?

                                                                    (66)
            Breathlessness 1
            Coughing 2
            Wheezing 3
            Get asthma/make asthma worse 4
            Prone to chest infections/bronchitis 5
            Likely to suffer from cancer 6
            Likely to suffer from another serious
              illness (SPECIFY & CODE 7)

            7
            Baby likely to be born small/underweight 8
            Baby likely to be born prematurely 9
            Baby likely to have chest health problems 0
            Baby less likely to grow X
            Other (WRITE IN & CODE Y)

            .... Y
                                                                    (67)
            Don't know 1   (66-67)

ASK ALL PARENTS OF CHILDREN UNDER 16 (SEE QQ2&4) OTHERS GO TO Q227
Q222 About how many hours a day on average do you think your children are exposed to cigarette smoke?

            ☐☐
                                                                    (68-69)

ASK PARENTS WHERE THERE IS A SMOKER IN HOUSEHOLD (AS ABOVE, IF ONE OR MORE CODE 1's AT Q195-196). OTHER PARENTS GO TO Q225
Q223 SHOWCARD WW(R) AGAIN How much, if at all, do you think the health of your child/children is affected by people smoking in the home?

                                                                    (70)
            A great deal 1
            A fair amount 2   ASK Q224
            Just a little 3
            Not at all 4
            Don't know 5   GO TO Q225   (70)

ASK IF CODES 1-3 AT Q223
Q224 And in what ways do you think people smoking in the home affects the health of your child/children?

                                                                    (71)
            Breathlessness 1
            Coughing 2
            Wheezing 3
            Get asthma/makes asthma worse 4
            Prone to chest infections/bronchitis 5
            Likely to suffer from cancer 6
            Likely to suffer from another serious
              illness (SPECIFY & CODE 7)

            7
            Less likely to grow well 8
            General poor health 9
            Glue ear 0
            Other (WRITE IN AND CODE X) ....

            X
            Don't know .... Y   (71)

55

ASK ALL PARENTS OF CHILDREN UNDER 16
Q225 **Do you think parental smoking makes children more likely to smoke, less likely to smoke or does it make no difference?**

	(72)
More likely	1
Less likely	2
No difference	3
It depends	4
Don't know	5

(72)

ASK PARENTS WHO SMOKE (YES AT Q174)
Q226 **Do you think the fact that you smoke makes your child/children more likely to smoke themselves, less likely to smoke or does it make no difference?**

	(73)
More likely	1
Less likely	2
No difference	3
It depends	4
Don't know	5

(73)

ASK ALL
Q227 **Apart from any visit to a hospital, when did you last talk to a doctor, either in person or by telephone, on your own behalf (that is about something to do with your own health)?**

	(74)
In last week	1
Over 1 week, within 2 weeks	2
Over 2 weeks, within last month	3
Over 1 month, within last 2 months	4
Over 2 months, within last 3 months	5
Over 3 months, within last 4 months	6
Over 4 months, within last 6 months	7
Over 6 months, within last 12 months	8
Over 1 year, within last 3 years	9
Over 3 years, within last 5 years	0
Over 5 years, within last 10 years	X
Over 10 years	Y
	(75)
Can't remember	1
Never	2

(74-75)

Q228 **And when did you last visit a doctor's or GP's surgery or a health centre on your own behalf? I am interested in any visit you may have made, not necessarily involving seeing the GP.**

	(76)
In last week	1
Over 1 week, within 2 weeks	2
Over 2 weeks, within last month	3
Over 1 month, within last 2 months	4
Over 2 months, within last 3 months	5
Over 3 months, within last 4 months	6
Over 4 months, within last 6 months	7
Over 6 months, within last 12 months	8
Over 1 year, within last 3 years	9
Over 3 years, within last 5 years	0
Over 5 years, within last 10 years	X
Over 10 years	Y
	(77)
Can't remember	1
Never	2

(76-77)

IF RESPONDENT IS AGED 16-54, NOW HAND OVER SEXUAL HEALTH QUESTIONNAIRE (MEN'S OR WOMEN'S VERSION AS APPROPRIATE). IF RESPONDENT IS AGED 55+, GO TO RESPONDENT FEEDBACK AFTER CODING BELOW. NB YOU SHOULD ALREADY HAVE STUCK A SERIAL NUMBERED LABEL TO THE BACK OF THIS QUESTIONNAIRE BUT JUST MAKE SURE IT IS THERE.

SAY:

> "This questionnaire is designed for you to complete on your own. Please read the instructions on the front page carefully and then try to answer the questions. I realise you may consider some of these questions very personal. They may concern matters that normally you do not discuss even with your partner or close friends. However, the Health Education Authority is trying to make sure that relevant health care is provided to all members of the community, and this is why we are asking people to let us have this information. HAND OVER BROWN ENVELOPE. When you have finished with the questionnaire, put it into the envelope, seal it and hand it back to me."

STRESS:
- ENTIRELY PRIVATE AND CONFIDENTIAL, NO NAME ON QUESTIONNAIRE
- SERIOUS PIECE OF SOCIAL RESEARCH WITH THE AIM OF PREVENTING UNNECESSARY ILLNESSES AND DEATHS

PLEASE RECORD BELOW THE RESPONSE TO THE SELF-COMPLETION QUESTIONNAIRE

                                                                            (78)
Questionnaire accepted 1
Questionnaire refused 2
Respondent aged 55+ 3
Respondent physically unable to complete it (eg poor sight, can't read) 4
Other (PLEASE WRITE IN AND CODE 5) 5
. . . . _____ (78)

IF QUESTIONNAIRE ACCEPTED, HOW LONG DID IT TAKE TO COMPLETE? (PLEASE TIME SEPARATELY FROM REST OF QUESTIONNAIRE)

WRITE IN ⬜⬜ MINUTES   (79-80)

                                                              CARD⑧   10

PLEASE COMPLETE THE FOLLOWING COMMENTS FOR ALL CODED 1 OR 2 ABOVE

1)   DID THE RESPONDENT ACTUALLY LOOK AT THE BACK OF THE QUESTIONNAIRE AT ALL?

                                                                      (11)
      Yes 1
      No 2

2)   DID THE RESPONDENT PAY ANY ATTENTION TO THE LABEL ON THE BACK OF THE QUESTIONNAIRE?

      Yes 3
      No 4

3)   IF THE RESPONDENT SAW THE LABEL, DID HE/SHE REACT TO IT IN ANY WAY (AS FAR AS YOU COULD SEE)?

      Yes (PLEASE DESCRIBE REACTION AND CODE 5) . . . .

      5

      No 6   (11)

Respondent Feedback

PLEASE COMPLETE THIS SECTION AT THE END OF THE INTERVIEW

I would like to end the interview by asking you what you thought about the interview.

Q229 **How interesting did you find the interview? Would you say . . . .**
READ OUT. ALTERNATE & TICK START

                                                (12)

☐   . . . **very interesting** 1
     . . . **fairly interesting** 2
     . . . **not very interesting** 3
☐   . . . **not at all interesting** 4
     Don't know 5   (12)

Q230 **And how long did you find the interview? Would you say . . . .**
READ OUT. ALTERNATE & TICK START

                                                (13)

☐   . . . **much too long** 1
     . . . **a little too long** 2
     . . . **about right** 3
☐   . . . **too short** 4
     Don't know 5   (13)

Q231 **Do you think the questions were difficult to understand or not? Would you say they were**
. . . . READ OUT. ALTERNATE & TICK START

                                                (14)

☐   . . . **very difficult** . . . . 1 ⎱ ASK Q232
     . . . **fairly difficult** . . . . 2 ⎰
     . . . **not very difficult** . . . . 3 ⎱ GO TO
☐   . . . **not at all difficult** . . . . 4 ⎱ Q233
     Don't know . . . . 5 ⎰ (14)

Q232 **Which questions did you find difficult?**

                                                (15)

Cholesterol/fats 1
Fat/fibre consumption 2
Cooking 3
Food buying 4
Smoking 5
Sexual Health 6
Other (WRITE IN & CODE 7)

. . . . 7
All of them 8
Don't know 9   (15)

58

Q233 **Finally, how interested would you be in participating in future surveys on similar subjects? Would you be . . . .**
READ OUT. ALTERNATE & TICK START

(16)

☐   . . . **very interested** 1
     . . . **fairly interested** 2
     . . . **not very interested** 3
     . . . **not at all interested** 4
☐   Don't know . . . . 5 _____ (16)

RECORD INTERVIEW LENGTH   ☐☐☐ minutes   (17-19)

THANK RESPONDENT & CLOSE

MORI/7191 **Health and Lifestyle Survey 1993**

C O N F I D E N T I A L

Self-Completion Section

MEN

Thank you very much for your help so far. The next set of questions are in this booklet and are of a more personal nature. It is probably easier for you to read them and tick the answers which apply to you.

It is very important that this survey provides a truly representative picture of the country as a whole. Therefore we need your responses to be as complete, honest and accurate as possible, even though the questions may not always seem relevant to you personally.

Please do not put your name anywhere on this questionnaire. When you have finished, put the questionnaire into the envelope and seal it before returning it to the interviewer. MORI will keep your answers in strictest confidence - the answers from everyone taking part in this survey will be analysed anonymously. We are very grateful for your help with this important project.

Q1 **Below are some statements about sex education. Please say how strongly you agree or disagree with each one.**
TICK ONE BOX FOR EACH STATEMENT

CARD (9) 10

	Strongly agree	Tend to agree	Tend to dis-agree	Strongly dis-agree	Don't know	
Sex education for young people should be provided mainly by parents	☐ 1	☐ 2	☐ 3	☐ 4	☐ 5	(11)
Schools are more important than parents when it comes to sex education for young people	☐ 1	☐ 2	☐ 3	☐ 4	☐ 5	(12)
Parents should be included by schools in helping with sex education for their children	☐ 1	☐ 2	☐ 3	☐ 4	☐ 5	(13)
Adverts about AIDS and condoms should not be shown on television before 9 pm	☐ 1	☐ 2	☐ 3	☐ 4	☐ 5	(14)
Most parents don't talk openly to their children about sexual matters	☐ 1	☐ 2	☐ 3	☐ 4	☐ 5	(15)

Q2 **For each of the following topics, please say how important you think it is that each one should or should not be included in sex education in schools.**
TICK ONE BOX FOR EACH TOPIC

	Very important to include	Fairly important to include	Fairly important not to include	Very important not to include	Don't know	
Human sexual reproduction	☐ 1	☐ 2	☐ 3	☐ 4	☐ 5	(16)
Contraception and family planning	☐ 1	☐ 2	☐ 3	☐ 4	☐ 5	(17)
How to use a condom	☐ 1	☐ 2	☐ 3	☐ 4	☐ 5	(18)
Homosexuality and lesbianism	☐ 1	☐ 2	☐ 3	☐ 4	☐ 5	(19)
How HIV (the AIDS virus) is passed on	☐ 1	☐ 2	☐ 3	☐ 4	☐ 5	(20)
How other sexually transmitted diseases are passed on	☐ 1	☐ 2	☐ 3	☐ 4	☐ 5	(21)
How to express feelings and emotions in sexual relationships	☐ 1	☐ 2	☐ 3	☐ 4	☐ 5	(22)
How to talk to sexual partners about safer sex	☐ 1	☐ 2	☐ 3	☐ 4	☐ 5	(23)
How to make personal choices about having sexual relationships	☐ 1	☐ 2	☐ 3	☐ 4	☐ 5	(24)

Q3 **Which of these items do you think you have adequate knowledge or information about?**
TICK ALL THE BOXES THAT APPLY

Contraception/birth control	☐ 1
Emergency ("morning after") contraception	☐ 2
Ways in which HIV (the AIDS virus) can be passed on	☐ 3
Ways in which other sexually transmitted diseases can be passed on	☐ 4
Recognising symptoms of sexually transmitted disease	☐ 5
Having a blood test for the AIDS virus (HIV test)	☐ 6
How to express your love/feelings to your partner	☐ 7
How to express better to a partner your sexual needs	☐ 8
How to satisfy the sexual needs of your partner	☐ 9
How to raise the subject of safer sex	☐ 0
None of these	☐ x

(25)

Q4 **Here are some ways in which you might describe your own sexual lifestyle. Whatever your sexual lifestyle - whether very sexually active, quite sexually active or not sexually active at all - please show how you would describe your sexual lifestyle most of the time these days.**
TICK ONE BOX IN EACH LINE FOR a), b), c) AND d)

These days my sexual lifestyle is . . . .

a) | **Very fulfilling** | **Quite fulfilling** | **Not very fulfilling** | **Not at all fulfilling** |
|---|---|---|---|
| ☐ 1 | ☐ 2 | ☐ 3 | ☐ 4 (26) |

b) | **Very exciting** | **Quite exciting** | **Not very exciting** | **Not at all exciting** |
|---|---|---|---|
| ☐ 1 | ☐ 2 | ☐ 3 | ☐ 4 (27) |

c) | **Exactly the way I would want it to be** | **Quite like the way I would want it to be** | **Not very much like the way I would want it to be** | **Not at all the way I would want it to be** (28) |
|---|---|---|---|
| ☐ 1 | ☐ 2 | ☐ 3 | ☐ 4 |

d) | **Completely under my control** | **Mainly under my control** | **A little under my control** | **Not at all under my control** |
|---|---|---|---|
| ☐ 1 | ☐ 2 | ☐ 3 | ☐ 4 (29) |

The next few questions are about the risks of HIV infection (the AIDS virus) and other sexually transmitted diseases.

Q5 What do you think are the chances on average these days, of people in this country getting HIV (the AIDS virus), from sexual intercourse without a condom between men and women?
TICK ONE BOX

Very high	☐ 1
Fairly high	☐ 2
Moderate	☐ 3
Fairly low	☐ 4
Very low	☐ 5
Don't know	☐ 6

(30)

Q6 With your present sexual lifestyle, how much at risk do you personally feel of becoming infected with HIV (the AIDS virus)?
TICK ONE BOX

Greatly at risk	☐ 1
Quite a lot at risk	☐ 2
Not very much at risk	☐ 3
Not at all at risk	☐ 4
Don't know	☐ 5

(31)

Q7 And with your present sexual lifestyle, how much at risk do you personally feel of becoming infected with other sexually transmitted diseases?
TICK ONE BOX

Greatly at risk	☐ 1
Quite a lot at risk	☐ 2
Not very much at risk	☐ 3
Not at all at risk	☐ 4
Don't know	☐ 5

(32)

Q8 Compared to other men of your age living in this country, do you feel that your chances of getting HIV (the AIDS virus) from vaginal sexual intercourse without a condom are .

TICK ONE BOX

Much less than average	☐ 1
Slightly less than average	☐ 2
About average	☐ 3
Slightly greater than average	☐ 4
Much greater than average	☐ 5
Don't know	☐ 6

(33)

Q9 And compared to other men of your age living in this country, do you feel that your chances of getting any other sexually transmitted disease are . . .
TICK ONE BOX

Much less than average	☐ 1
Slightly less than average	☐ 2
About average	☐ 3
Slightly greater than average	☐ 4
Much greater than average	☐ 5
Don't know	☐ 6

(34)

Q10 How strongly do you agree or disagree with the following statements?
TICK ONE BOX FOR EACH STATEMENT

	Strongly agree	Tend to agree	Tend to disagree	Strongly disagree	Don't know	
I don't think I'll ever get HIV (the AIDs virus)	☐ 1	☐ 2	☐ 3	☐ 4	☐ 5	(35)
For me, risky sex is better than no sex	☐ 1	☐ 2	☐ 3	☐ 4	☐ 5	(36)
Getting HIV (the AIDS virus) is something that worries me about my sexual lifestyle these days	☐ 1	☐ 2	☐ 3	☐ 4	☐ 5	(37)

The next few questions are about your own sexual experiences.

Q11   **How old were you when you <u>first</u> had sexual intercourse with a woman?**
WRITE IN THE AGE IN THE BOXES

☐☐ years   (38-39)

If this has not happened to you yet, tick this box ☐ and go on to Q35 on page 17   (39/Y)

Q12   **Did you or your partner use any form of contraception or take any precautions that <u>first</u> time, or not?**
TICK ALL THE BOXES THAT APPLY

The pill	☐ 1
The female condom	☐ 2
Condom/sheath/Durex	☐ 3
Other contraception	☐ 4
I withdrew	☐ 5
Made sure it was a "safe period"	☐ 6
No precautions by me, don't know about partner	☐ 7
No precautions by either of us	☐ 8
Can't remember	☐ 9
Don't know	☐ 0	(40)

Q13   **How long ago did you <u>last</u> have sexual intercourse with a woman?**
TICK ONE BOX

Within the last week	☐ 1
Within the last 2 weeks	☐ 2
Within the last 3 weeks	☐ 3
Within the last 4 weeks	☐ 4
Within the last 6 weeks	☐ 5
Within the last 3 months	☐ 6
Within the last 6 months	☐ 7
Within the last 9 months	☐ 8
Within the last 12 months	☐ 9
Within the last 2 years	☐ 0
Within the last 5 years	☐ x
5 years ago or more	☐ Y
Cannot remember	☐ 1	(41-42)

Q14   **At the time you last had sexual intercourse, for how long had you been in a sexual relationship with this woman?**
TICK ONE BOX

Less than 12 hours	☐ 1
Less than 1 week	☐ 2
Less than 4 weeks	☐ 3
Less than 3 months	☐ 4
Less than 6 months	☐ 5
Less than 12 months	☐ 6
Less than 2 years	☐ 7
Less than 5 years	☐ 8
Less than 10 years	☐ 9
Less than 20 years	☐ 0
20 years or more	☐ x
Cannot remember	☐ y

(43)

Q15   **And at the time you last had sexual intercourse, for how long had you known this woman altogether, that is including any period before starting a sexual relationship?**
TICK ONE BOX

Less than 12 hours	☐ 1
Less than 1 week	☐ 2
Less than 4 weeks	☐ 3
Less than 3 months	☐ 4
Less than 6 months	☐ 5
Less than 12 months	☐ 6
Less than 2 years	☐ 7
Less than 5 years	☐ 8
Less than 10 years	☐ 9
Less than 20 years	☐ 0
20 years or more	☐ x
Cannot remember	☐ y

(44)

Q16 **When you last had sexual intercourse, what kind of relationship were you in with this woman? Were you . . . .**
TICK ONE BOX

Married to each other	☐ 1
Living together (not married)	☐ 2
Steady partners (not living together)	☐ 3
Not steady partners at the time	☐ 4
Can't remember	☐ 5

(45)

Q17 **When you last had sexual intercourse with a woman, which of these if any were used? (More than one may have been used, so please tick all that apply.)**

The pill	☐ 1
Emergency ("morning after") contraception	☐ 2
The coil/IUD/intra-uterine device	☐ 3
The female condom	☐ 4
Condom/sheath/Durex	☐ 5
Cap/diaphragm/Dutch cap	☐ 6
Foam tablets/jellies/creams	☐ 7
Suppositories/pessaries/aerosol foam	☐ 8
Sponge	☐ 9
Douching/washing	☐ 0
Safe period/rhythm method	☐ x
Withdrawal	☐ Y
Sterilisation/vasectomy	☐ 1
Other method of protection	☐ 2

. . . .

None	☐ 3
Can't remember	☐ 4

(46-47)

PLEASE ANSWER THE NEXT 3 QUESTIONS IF YOU TICKED THE BOX FOR "CONDOM" OR "FEMALE CONDOM" AT Q17. (IF NOT, PLEASE GO TO Q21a ON PAGE 12)

Q18 **If a <u>condom</u> was used on this last occasion of sexual intercourse, please say what was the <u>main</u> reason.**
TICK ONE BOX

For contraception	☐ 1
For protection against HIV (the AIDS virus)	☐ 2
For protection against other sexually transmitted diseases	☐ 3
Other reason	☐ 4
Can't remember/don't know	☐ 5

(48)

Q19 **And what if any was <u>another</u> reason for using a condom?**
TICK ALL THE BOXES THAT APPLY

For contraception	☐ 1
For protection against HIV (the AIDS virus)	☐ 2
For protection against other sexually transmitted diseases	☐ 3
Other reason	☐ 4
Can't remember/don't know	☐ 5

(49)

Q20 **And who suggested using a condom?**

Your suggestion	☐ 1	
Your partner's suggestion	☐ 2	
Both	☐ 3	NOW GO TO Q22
Didn't talk about it	☐ 4	
Can't remember	☐ 5	

(50)

PLEASE ANSWER Q21 IF YOU DID NOT TICK 'CONDOM' OR 'FEMALE CONDOM' AT Q17

Q21a) **If you did not use a condom on the last occasion you had sexual intercourse with a woman, what was the main reason for this?** PLEASE WRITE IN (51)

_____

_____ (52)

_____

b) **And what (if anything) was another reason for not using a condom?** PLEASE WRITE IN (53)

_____

_____ (54)

_____

- 13 -

EVERYONE PLEASE ANSWER Q22

Q22 In the last 12 months, with how many women have you had vaginal sexual intercourse?
Please include every woman you have had vaginal sexual intercourse within the last 12
months, even if only once. Please remember to include your present partner (if you
have had vaginal sexual intercourse with her). If you can't remember exactly please
give your best estimate.

Number of partners	TICK ONE BOX		
None	☐ 0	13	☐ 2
1	☐ 1	14	☐ 3
2	☐ 2	15	☐ 4
3	☐ 3	16	☐ 5
4	☐ 4	17	☐ 6
5	☐ 5	18	☐ 7
6	☐ 6	19	☐ 8
7	☐ 7	20	☐ 9
8	☐ 8	21-25	☐ 0
9	☐ 9	26-30	☐ x
10	☐ x	31-40	☐ y
11	☐ y	41-50	☐ 1
12	☐ 1	51-100	☐ 2
		More than 100	☐ 3

(53-57)

Q23   Below is a list of different kinds of sexual contact. Please indicate for each one whether or not you have had this kind of sexual contact <u>over the last 12 months.</u>

Q24   And for each kind of sexual contact you have had, please write in the boxes provided the number of different women with whom you had this kind of contact over the last 12 months. Remember to include your current partner if appropriate.

	Q23 In last 12 months		Q24 Number of women	
	No	Yes		

Oral sex on man by woman
(woman's mouth on man's genital area)

a)   without a condom   ☐₁   ☐₂   ☐☐ women   (58-60)

b)   with a condom   ☐₁   ☐₂   ☐☐ women   (61-63)

Oral sex on woman by man

(man's mouth on woman's genital area)   ☐₁   ☐₂   ☐☐ women   (64-66)

Vaginal intercourse
(man's penis entering woman's vagina)

a)   without a condom   ☐₁   ☐₂   ☐☐ women   (67-69)

b)   with a condom   ☐₁   ☐₂   ☐☐ women   (70-72)

Anal intercourse
(man's penis entering woman's anus/back passage)

a)   without a condom   ☐₁   ☐₂   ☐☐ women   (73-75)

b)   with a condom   ☐₁   ☐₂   ☐☐ women   (76-78)

CARD ⑩   10

Q25   Altogether, what is the total number of different women with whom you have had any of the above kinds of sexual contact, over the last 12 months?   Please remember to include your present partner if appropriate.

WRITE THE NUMBER IN THE BOXES PROVIDED

☐☐☐ partners   (11-13)

(IF NONE, WRITE '000' IN THE BOXES AND GO TO Q28 OVERLEAF)

Q26 **Thinking of the occasions when you had sexual intercourse in the last 12 months, how often did you use condoms?**
TICK ONE BOX

Always	☐ 1
Most times	☐ 2
About half the time	☐ 3
Occasionally	☐ 4
Never	☐ 5

(14)

Q27 **Now thinking just of the occasions when you have had sexual intercourse with any new partners within the last 12 months, how often did you use a condom?**
TICK ONE BOX

Not had any new partners in last 12 months	☐ 1
Always	☐ 2
Most times	☐ 3
About half the time	☐ 4
Occasionally	☐ 5
Never	☐ 6

(15)

Q28 **Do you intend to use condoms in the next 12 months?**
TICK ONE BOX

Definitely	☐ 1
Probably	☐ 2
Probably not	☐ 3
Definitely not	☐ 4

(16)

Q29 **Have you ever gone on your own initiative to have a blood test for the AIDS virus (HIV test)?**
TICK ONE BOX

No	☐ 1	NOW GO TO Q35
Yes	☐ 2	ANSWER Q30-34

(17)

Q30 **If yes, when was that test? (The last HIV test you have had if more than one.)**
TICK ONE BOX

In the last 12 months	☐ 1
Between 1 and 2 years ago	☐ 2
More than 2 years ago	☐ 3
Can't remember	☐ 4

(18)

Q31 **Why did you go for this HIV test?**
TICK ALL THE BOXES THAT APPLY

Have been at risk of infection through
sexual contact abroad □ 1
Have been at risk of infection through
sexual contact in this country □ 2
Have been at risk of infection through
injecting drug use □ 3

Other reason (PLEASE TICK BOX AND WRITE IN)

. . . . □ 4   (19)

Q32 **And where did you have that test?**
TICK ONE BOX

Blood donor centre □ 1
Ante-natal clinic □ 2
Other hospital department/clinic □ 3
Private doctor or private clinic □ 4
GP or family doctor's surgery/health centre □ 5
STD or VD clinic □ 6
Somewhere else (PLEASE TICK BOX AND WRITE IN WHERE)

. . . . □ 7   (20)

Q33 **Did you receive the results of this test?**
TICK ONE BOX

No   □ 1   NOW GO TO Q35
Yes   □ 2   ANSWER Q34   (21)

Q34 **How helpful was any counselling you received concerning the HIV test?**
TICK ONE BOX

Did not get any
counselling   □ 1
Not at all helpful   □ 2
Not very helpful   □ 3
Fairly helpful   □ 4
Very helpful   □ 5   (22)

EVERYONE PLEASE ANSWER Q35
Q35 **Which of the following applies to you?**
TICK ONE BOX

I have had sexual experience only with females
(or a female), never with a male   ☐ 1

I have had sexual experience more often with females,
and at least once with a male   ☐ 2

I have had sexual experience about equally often with
males and with females   ☐ 3

I have had sexual experience more often with males,
and at least once with a female   ☐ 4

I have had sexual experience only with males
(or a male), never with a female   ☐ 5

I have never had any sexual experience with anyone   ☐ 6   (23)

IF YOU HAVE NEVER HAD ANY SEXUAL EXPERIENCE WITH ANYONE,
PLEASE DO NOT ANSWER ANY FURTHER QUESTIONS (THANKS FOR
YOUR HELP). EVERYONE ELSE PLEASE CONTINUE WITH THE
QUESTIONNAIRE.

Q36 **Have you ever had sex with a male involving genital area/penis contact?**
TICK ONE BOX

No   ☐ 1 GO TO Q38
Yes   ☐ 2 ANSWER Q37   (24)

Q37 **If yes, when was the last occasion?**
TICK ONE BOX

Within the last 4 weeks   ☐ 1
Between 4 weeks and 3 months ago   ☐ 2
Between 3 months and 6 months ago   ☐ 3
Between 6 months and 1 year ago   ☐ 4
Between 1 year and 5 years ago   ☐ 5
More than 5 years ago   ☐ 6   (25)

We would now like to ask some questions about your attitudes to condoms. Please remember that we do need your responses to these questions, to ensure that we get a representative picture for the whole range of people in this country.

Q38 Listed below are some advantages and disadvantages which people have mentioned about using condoms. Thinking of your own sexual lifestyle and sexual partner(s), please tick one box next to each statement to show how likely or unlikely you think it would be in your case.

TICK ONE BOX FOR EACH STATEMENT

	Very unlikely	Fairly unlikely	Fairly likely	Very likely	
Using condoms would...					
...make sex less enjoyable for me	☐ 1	☐ 2	☐ 3	☐ 4	(26)
...protect against unwanted pregnancy	☐ 1	☐ 2	☐ 3	☐ 4	(27)
...make sex less romantic	☐ 1	☐ 2	☐ 3	☐ 4	(28)
...protect against being infected with HIV (the AIDS virus)	☐ 1	☐ 2	☐ 3	☐ 4	(29)
...protect against being infected with other sexually transmitted diseases (STDs)	☐ 1	☐ 2	☐ 3	☐ 4	(30)
...show that I was a caring person	☐ 1	☐ 2	☐ 3	☐ 4	(31)
...make sex less spontaneous	☐ 1	☐ 2	☐ 3	☐ 4	(32)
...cause offence to my partner	☐ 1	☐ 2	☐ 3	☐ 4	(33)
...make my partner think that I might be infected with HIV	☐ 1	☐ 2	☐ 3	☐ 4	(34)
...make me feel less of a man	☐ 1	☐ 2	☐ 3	☐ 4	(35)
...give my partner the impression that I sleep around	☐ 1	☐ 2	☐ 3	☐ 4	(36)
...make sex messy	☐ 1	☐ 2	☐ 3	☐ 4	(37)
...reduce my sexual pleasure	☐ 1	☐ 2	☐ 3	☐ 4	(38)
...reduce my partner's sexual pleasure	☐ 1	☐ 2	☐ 3	☐ 4	(39)
...be an annoying interruption to sex	☐ 1	☐ 2	☐ 3	☐ 4	(40)
...make sex embarrassing	☐ 1	☐ 2	☐ 3	☐ 4	(41)
...be difficult to plan ahead for	☐ 1	☐ 2	☐ 3	☐ 4	(42)

Q39 And how much do you care about...
TICK ONE BOX FOR EACH STATEMENT

	Not at all	A little	A lot	
...sex being less enjoyable for you	☐ 1	☐ 2	☐ 3	(43)
...protecting against unwanted pregnancy	☐ 1	☐ 2	☐ 3	(44)
...sex being less romantic	☐ 1	☐ 2	☐ 3	(45)
...protecting against being infected with HIV	☐ 1	☐ 2	☐ 3	(46)
...protecting against being infected with other sexually transmitted diseases	☐ 1	☐ 2	☐ 3	(47)
...showing that you are a caring person	☐ 1	☐ 2	☐ 3	(48)
...sex being less spontaneous	☐ 1	☐ 2	☐ 3	(49)
...causing offence to your partner	☐ 1	☐ 2	☐ 3	(50)
...your partner thinking that you might be infected with HIV	☐ 1	☐ 2	☐ 3	(51)
...feeling less of a man	☐ 1	☐ 2	☐ 3	(52)
...giving your partner the impression that you sleep around	☐ 1	☐ 2	☐ 3	(53)
...sex being messy	☐ 1	☐ 2	☐ 3	(54)
...your sexual pleasure being reduced	☐ 1	☐ 2	☐ 3	(55)
...your partner's sexual pleasure being reduced	☐ 1	☐ 2	☐ 3	(56)
...having an annoying interruption to sex	☐ 1	☐ 2	☐ 3	(57)
...sex being embarrassing	☐ 1	☐ 2	☐ 3	(58)
...having to plan ahead for sex	☐ 1	☐ 2	☐ 3	(59)

Q40   Listed below are some statements about the views and behaviour of other people.
Again, thinking of your sexual lifestyle and sexual partner(s), please tick a box to
indicate how much you agree or disagree with each statement.
TICK ONE BOX FOR EACH STATEMENT

	Strongly agree	Tend to agree	Tend to disagree	Strongly disagree	
My current sexual partner thinks we should use condoms	□₁	□₂	□₃	□₄	(80)
A new sexual partner would want me to use condoms	□₁	□₂	□₃	□₄	(81)
My friends would approve if I used condoms	□₁	□₂	□₃	□₄	(82)
My doctor would approve if I used condoms	□₁	□₂	□₃	□₄	(83)
Government health campaigns recommend that I use condoms	□₁	□₂	□₃	□₄	(84)
Most people who are important to me would approve if I used condoms	□₁	□₂	□₃	□₄	(85)

Q41   In general ...
TICK ONE BOX FOR EACH STATEMENT

	Strongly agree	Tend to agree	Tend to disagree	Strongly disagree	
I would want to do what my current sexual partner thinks I should do	□₁	□₂	□₃	□₄	(66)
I would want to do what a new sexual partner wanted me to do	□₁	□₂	□₃	□₄	(67)
I would want to do what my friends wanted me to do	□₁	□₂	□₃	□₄	(68)
I would want to do what my doctor wanted me to do	□₁	□₂	□₃	□₄	(69)
I would want to do what Government health campaigns recommended me to do	□₁	□₂	□₃	□₄	(70)

Q42 **How likely is it that each of the following would stop you using condoms, even if you wished to use them?**

TICK ONE BOX FOR EACH STATEMENT

	Very unlikely	Fairly unlikely	Fairly likely	Very likely	
Feeling embarrassed to buy condoms	☐ 1	☐ 2	☐ 3	☐ 4	(71)
Forgetting to carry them with you	☐ 1	☐ 2	☐ 3	☐ 4	(72)
Difficulty in using a condom	☐ 1	☐ 2	☐ 3	☐ 4	(73)
The cost of condoms	☐ 1	☐ 2	☐ 3	☐ 4	(74)
Difficulty in obtaining condoms	☐ 1	☐ 2	☐ 3	☐ 4	(75)
Getting carried away in the heat of the moment	☐ 1	☐ 2	☐ 3	☐ 4	(76)
Difficulty in talking about using condoms	☐ 1	☐ 2	☐ 3	☐ 4	(77)
Your partner getting angry if you suggested using condoms	☐ 1	☐ 2	☐ 3	☐ 4	(78)
Fear of giving a bad impression about your own sexual behaviour if you suggested using condoms	☐ 1	☐ 2	☐ 3	☐ 4	(79)
Difficulty in planning ahead for sex	☐ 1	☐ 2	☐ 3	☐ 4	(80)

CARD (11)   10

Q43 **How strongly do you agree or disagree with each of these statements?**
TICK ONE BOX FOR EACH STATEMENT

	Strongly agree	Tend to agree	Tend to disagree	Strongly disagree	
For me, the disadvantages of using condoms would outweigh the advantages	☐ 1	☐ 2	☐ 3	☐ 4	(11)
For me, using condoms would be a good idea	☐ 1	☐ 2	☐ 3	☐ 4	(12)
Most people whose opinions I value think I should use condoms	☐ 1	☐ 2	☐ 3	☐ 4	(13)
I intend to use condoms in the future	☐ 1	☐ 2	☐ 3	☐ 4	(14)
More and more people are using condoms these days	☐ 1	☐ 2	☐ 3	☐ 4	(15)
More and more of my friends are using condoms these days	☐ 1	☐ 2	☐ 3	☐ 4	(16)

Q44   How much control do you have over whether or not you use condoms?
TICK ONE BOX

Complete control	A lot of control	Some control	Very little control	
☐ 1	☐ 2	☐ 3	☐ 4	(17)

Q45   How easy or difficult would it be for you to do each of the following, if you wanted to?
TICK ONE BOX FOR EACH ITEM

	Very easy	Fairly easy	Fairly difficult	Very difficult	
Choose sexual partners that were not at risk of infection	☐ 1	☐ 2	☐ 3	☐ 4	(18)
Use condoms with a sexual partner	☐ 1	☐ 2	☐ 3	☐ 4	(19)
Persuade a sexual partner to have sex with a condom if they didn't want to	☐ 1	☐ 2	☐ 3	☐ 4	(20)

Thinking of the next 12 months . . . .

Q46   How likely is it that you will use condoms in the next 12 months?
       TICK ONE BOX

Very unlikely	Fairly unlikely	Fairly likely	Very likely	
☐ 1	☐ 2	☐ 3	☐ 4	(21)

Q47   Thinking of the occasions when you may have sexual intercourse in the next 12 months, how often do you think you will use condoms?
       TICK ONE BOX

Always	Most times	About half the time	Occasionally	Never	
☐ 1	☐ 2	☐ 3	☐ 4	☐ 5	(22)

Q48   How likely is it that you would use condoms if you had sex with a new partner?
       TICK ONE BOX

Very unlikely	Fairly unlikely	Fairly likely	Very likely	
☐ 1	☐ 2	☐ 3	☐ 4	(23)

Q49   Thinking just of the occasions when you may have sexual intercourse with any new partners in the next 12 months, how often do you think you will use condoms?
       TICK ONE BOX

Always	Most times	About half the time	Occasionally	Never	
☐ 1	☐ 2	☐ 3	☐ 4	☐ 5	(24)

THANK YOU VERY MUCH FOR COMPLETING THIS QUESTIONNAIRE

YOUR ANSWERS WILL BE KEPT IN COMPLETE CONFIDENCE

MORI/7191

Health and Lifestyle Survey 1993

C O N F I D E N T I A L

Self-Completion Section

WOMEN

Thank you very much for your help so far. The next set of questions are in this booklet and are of a more personal nature. It is probably easier for you to read them and tick the answers which apply to you.

It is very important that this survey provides a truly representative picture of the country as a whole. Therefore we need your responses to be as complete, honest and accurate as possible, even though the questions may not always seem relevant to you personally.

Please do not put your name anywhere on this questionnaire. When you have finished, put the questionnaire into the envelope and seal it before returning it to the interviewer. MORI will keep your answers in strictest confidence - the answers from everyone taking part in this survey will be analysed anonymously. We are very grateful for your help with this important project.

Q1 **Below are some statements about sex education. Please say how strongly you agree or disagree with each one.**
TICK ONE BOX FOR EACH STATEMENT

CARD (9) 1(

	Strongly agree	Tend to agree	Tend to dis-agree	Strongly dis-agree	Don't know	
Sex education for young people should be provided mainly by parents	□ 1	□ 2	□ 3	□ 4	□ 5	(11)
Schools are more important than parents when it comes to sex education for young people	□ 1	□ 2	□ 3	□ 4	□ 5	(12)
Parents should be included by schools in helping with sex education for their children	□ 1	□ 2	□ 3	□ 4	□ 5	(13)
Adverts about AIDS and condoms should not be shown on television before 9 pm	□ 1	□ 2	□ 3	□ 4	□ 5	(14)
Most parents don't talk openly to their children about sexual matters	□ 1	□ 2	□ 3	□ 4	□ 5	(15)

Q2 **For each of the following topics, please say how important you think it is that each one should or should not be included in sex education in schools.**
TICK ONE BOX FOR EACH TOPIC

	Very important to include	Fairly important to include	Fairly important not to include	Very important not to include	Don't know	
Human sexual reproduction	□ 1	□ 2	□ 3	□ 4	□ 5	(16)
Contraception and family planning	□ 1	□ 2	□ 3	□ 4	□ 5	(17)
How to use a condom	□ 1	□ 2	□ 3	□ 4	□ 5	(18)
Homosexuality and lesbianism	□ 1	□ 2	□ 3	□ 4	□ 5	(19)
How HIV (the AIDS virus) is passed on	□ 1	□ 2	□ 3	□ 4	□ 5	(20)
How other sexually transmitted diseases are passed on	□ 1	□ 2	□ 3	□ 4	□ 5	(21)
How to express feelings and emotions in sexual relationships	□ 1	□ 2	□ 3	□ 4	□ 5	(22)
How to talk to sexual partners about safer sex	□ 1	□ 2	□ 3	□ 4	□ 5	(23)
How to make personal choices about having sexual relationships	□ 1	□ 2	□ 3	□ 4	□ 5	(24)

Q3 **Which of these items do you think you have adequate knowledge or information about?**
TICK ALL THE BOXES THAT APPLY

Contraception/birth control   ☐ ₁

Emergency ("morning after") contraception   ☐ ₂

Ways in which HIV (the AIDS virus) can be passed on   ☐ ₃

Ways in which other sexually transmitted diseases
  can be passed on   ☐ ₄

Recognising symptoms of sexually transmitted disease   ☐ ₅

Having a blood test for the AIDS virus (HIV test)   ☐ ₆

How to express your love/feelings to your partner   ☐ ₇

How to express better to a partner your sexual needs   ☐ ₈

How to satisfy the sexual needs of your partner   ☐ ₉

How to raise the subject of safer sex   ☐ ₀

None of these   ☐ ₓ   (25)

Q4   Here are some ways in which you might describe your own sexual lifestyle. Whatever your sexual lifestyle - whether very sexually active, quite sexually active or not sexually active at all - please show how you would describe your sexual lifestyle most of the time these days.
TICK ONE BOX IN EACH LINE FOR a), b), c) AND d)

These days my sexual lifestyle is . . . .

a)   **Very fulfilling**   **Quite fulfilling**   **Not very fulfilling**   **Not at all fulfilling**

☐ 1   ☐ 2   ☐ 3   ☐ 4   (26)

b)   **Very exciting**   **Quite exciting**   **Not very exciting**   **Not at all exciting**

☐ 1   ☐ 2   ☐ 3   ☐ 4   (27)

c)   **Exactly the way I would want it to be**   **Quite like the way I would want it to be**   **Not very much like the way I would want it to be**   **Not at all the way I would want it to be**

☐ 1   ☐ 2   ☐ 3   ☐ 4   (28)

d)   **Completely under my control**   **Mainly under my control**   **A little under my control**   **Not at all under my control**

☐ 1   ☐ 2   ☐ 3   ☐ 4   (29)

The next few questions are about the risks of HIV infection (the AIDS virus) and other sexually transmitted diseases.

Q5   **What do you think are the chances on average these days, of people in this country getting HIV (the AIDS virus), from sexual intercourse without a condom between men and women?**
TICK ONE BOX

Very high	☐	1
Fairly high	☐	2
Moderate	☐	3
Fairly low	☐	4
Very low	☐	5
Don't know	☐	6

(30)

Q6   **With your present sexual lifestyle, how much at risk do you personally feel of becoming infected with HIV (the AIDS virus)?**
TICK ONE BOX

Greatly at risk	☐	1
Quite a lot at risk	☐	2
Not very much at risk	☐	3
Not at all at risk	☐	4
Don't know	☐	5

(31)

Q7   **And with your present sexual lifestyle, how much at risk do you personally feel of becoming infected with other sexually transmitted diseases?**
TICK ONE BOX

Greatly at risk	☐	1
Quite a lot at risk	☐	2
Not very much at risk	☐	3
Not at all at risk	☐	4
Don't know	☐	5

(32)

Q8 **Compared to other women of your age living in this country, do you feel that your chances of getting HIV (the AIDS virus) from vaginal sexual intercourse without a condom are . .**
TICK ONE BOX

Much less than average	☐ 1
Slightly less than average	☐ 2
About average	☐ 3
Slightly greater than average	☐ 4
Much greater than average	☐ 5
Don't know	☐ 6

(33)

Q9 **And compared to other women of your age living in this country, do you feel that your chances of getting any other sexually transmitted disease are . . .**
TICK ONE BOX

Much less than average	☐ 1
Slightly less than average	☐ 2
About average	☐ 3
Slightly greater than average	☐ 4
Much greater than average	☐ 5
Don't know	☐ 6

(34)

Q10 **How strongly do you agree or disagree with the following statements?**
TICK ONE BOX FOR EACH STATEMENT

	Strongly agree	Tend to agree	Tend to disagree	Strongly disagree	Don't know	
I don't think I'll ever get HIV (the AIDs virus)	☐ 1	☐ 2	☐ 3	☐ 4	☐ 5	(35)
For me, risky sex is better than no sex	☐ 1	☐ 2	☐ 3	☐ 4	☐ 5	(36)
Getting HIV (the AIDS virus) is something that worries me about my sexual lifestyle these days	☐ 1	☐ 2	☐ 3	☐ 4	☐ 5	(37)

The next few questions are about your own sexual experiences.

Q11   **How old were you when you <u>first</u> had sexual intercourse with a man?**
WRITE IN THE AGE IN THE BOXES

□□ years   (38-39)

If this has not happened to you yet, tick this box □ and go on to Q35 on page 17   (39/Y)

Q12   **Did you or your partner use any form of contraception or take any precautions that <u>first</u> time, or not?**
TICK ALL THE BOXES THAT APPLY

The pill	□ 1
The female condom	□ 2
Condom/sheath/Durex	□ 3
Other contraception	□ 4
He withdrew	□ 5
Made sure it was a "safe period"	□ 6
No precautions by me, don't know about partner	□ 7
No precautions by either of us	□ 8
Can't remember	□ 9
Don't know	□ 0

(40)

Q13   **How long ago did you <u>last</u> have sexual intercourse with a man?**
TICK ONE BOX

Within the last week	□ 1
Within the last 2 weeks	□ 2
Within the last 3 weeks	□ 3
Within the last 4 weeks	□ 4
Within the last 6 weeks	□ 5
Within the last 3 months	□ 6
Within the last 6 months	□ 7
Within the last 9 months	□ 8
Within the last 12 months	□ 9
Within the last 2 years	□ 0
Within the last 5 years	□ x
5 years ago or more	□ Y
Cannot remember	□ 1

(41-42)

Q14 **At the time you last had sexual intercourse, for how long had you been in a sexual relationship with this man?**
TICK ONE BOX

Less than 12 hours	☐ 1
Less than 1 week	☐ 2
Less than 4 weeks	☐ 3
Less than 3 months	☐ 4
Less than 6 months	☐ 5
Less than 12 months	☐ 6
Less than 2 years	☐ 7
Less than 5 years	☐ 8
Less than 10 years	☐ 9
Less than 20 years	☐ 0
20 years or more	☐ x
Cannot remember	☐ y	(43)

Q15 **And at the time you last had sexual intercourse, for how long had you known this man altogether, that is including any period before starting a sexual relationship?**
TICK ONE BOX

Less than 12 hours	☐ 1
Less than 1 week	☐ 2
Less than 4 weeks	☐ 3
Less than 3 months	☐ 4
Less than 6 months	☐ 5
Less than 12 months	☐ 6
Less than 2 years	☐ 7
Less than 5 years	☐ 8
Less than 10 years	☐ 9
Less than 20 years	☐ 0
20 years or more	☐ x
Cannot remember	☐ y	(44)

Q16 **When you last had sexual intercourse, what kind of relationship were you in with this man? Were you . . . .**
TICK ONE BOX

Married to each other	☐ 1
Living together (not married)	☐ 2
Steady partners (not living together)	☐ 3
Not steady partners at the time	☐ 4
Can't remember	☐ 5

(45)

Q17 **When you last had sexual intercourse with a man, which of these if any were used? (More than one may have been used, so please tick all that apply.)**

The pill	☐ 1
Emergency ("morning after") contraception	☐ 2
The coil/IUD/intra-uterine device	☐ 3
The female condom	☐ 4
Condom/sheath/Durex	☐ 5
Cap/diaphragm/Dutch cap	☐ 6
Foam tablets/jellies/creams	☐ 7
Suppositories/pessaries/aerosol foam	☐ 8
Sponge	☐ 9
Douching/washing	☐ 0
Safe period/rhythm method	☐ x
Withdrawal	☐ Y
Sterilisation/vasectomy	☐ 1
Other method of protection	☐ 2

. . . .

None	☐ 3
Can't remember	☐ 4

(46-47)

PLEASE ANSWER THE NEXT 3 QUESTIONS IF YOU TICKED THE BOX FOR 'CONDOM' OR 'FEMALE CONDOM' AT Q17. (IF NOT, PLEASE GO TO Q21a ON PAGE 12)

Q18 **If a <u>condom</u> was used on this last occasion of sexual intercourse, please say what was the <u>main</u> reason.**
TICK ONE BOX

For contraception	☐ 1	
For protection against HIV (the AIDS virus)	☐ 2	
For protection against other sexually transmitted diseases	☐ 3	
Other reason	☐ 4	
Can't remember/don't know	☐ 5	(48)

Q19 **And what if any was <u>another</u> reason for using a condom?**
TICK ALL THE BOXES THAT APPLY

For contraception	☐ 1	
For protection against HIV (the AIDS virus)	☐ 2	
For protection against other sexually transmitted diseases	☐ 3	
Other reason	☐ 4	
Can't remember/don't know	☐ 5	(49)

Q20 **And who suggested using a condom?**

Your suggestion	☐ 1	
Your partner's suggestion	☐ 2	
Both	☐ 3	NOW GO TO Q22
Didn't talk about it	☐ 4	
Can't remember	☐ 5	(50)

PLEASE ANSWER Q21 IF YOU DID NOT TICK 'CONDOM' OR 'FEMALE CONDOM' AT Q17

Q21a) **If you did not use a condom on the last occasion you had sexual intercourse with a man, what was the <u>main</u> reason for this? PLEASE WRITE IN** (51)

_____ (52)

_____

b) **And what (if anything) was another reason for not using a condom?** (53)
PLEASE WRITE IN

_____ (54)

_____

- 13 -

EVERYONE PLEASE ANSWER Q22

Q22   In the last 12 months, with how many men have you had vaginal sexual intercourse? Please include every man you have had vaginal sexual intercourse within the last 12 months, even if only once. Please remember to include your present partner (if you have had vaginal sexual intercourse with him). If you can't remember exactly please give your best estimate.

Number of partners   TICK ONE BOX

Number	Box	Number	Box
None	☐ 0	13	☐ 2
1	☐ 1	14	☐ 3
2	☐ 2	15	☐ 4
3	☐ 3	16	☐ 5
4	☐ 4	17	☐ 6
5	☐ 5	18	☐ 7
6	☐ 6	19	☐ 8
7	☐ 7	20	☐ 9
8	☐ 8	21-25	☐ 0
9	☐ 9	26-30	☐ x
10	☐ x	31-40	☐ Y
11	☐ Y	41-50	☐ 1
12	☐ 1	51-100	☐ 2
		More than 100	☐ 3

(55-57)

Q23   Below is a list of different kinds of sexual contact. Please indicate for each one whether or not you have had this kind of sexual contact <u>over the last 12 months.</u>

Q24   And for each kind of sexual contact you have had, please write in the boxes provided the number of different men with whom you had this kind of contact over the last 12 months. Remember to include your current partner if appropriate.

	Q23 In last 12 months No Yes	Q24 Number of men	
Oral sex on man by woman (woman's mouth on man's genital area)			
a) without a condom	☐₁ ☐₂	☐☐ men	(58-60)
b) with a condom	☐₁ ☐₂	☐☐ men	(61-63)
Oral sex on woman by man (man's mouth on woman's genital area)	☐₁ ☐₂	☐☐ men	(64-66)
Vaginal intercourse (man's penis entering woman's vagina)			
a) without a condom	☐₁ ☐₂	☐☐ men	(67-69)
b) with a condom	☐₁ ☐₂	☐☐ men	(70-72)
Anal intercourse (man's penis entering woman's anus/back passage)			
a) without a condom	☐₁ ☐₂	☐☐ men	(73-75)
b) with a condom	☐₁ ☐₂	☐☐ men	(76-78)

CARD 10

Q25   Altogether, what is the total number of different men with whom you have had any of the above kinds of sexual contact over the last 12 months? Please remember to include your present partner if appropriate.

WRITE THE NUMBER IN THE BOXES PROVIDED

☐☐☐ partners   (11-13)

(IF NONE, WRITE 000 IN THE BOXES AND GO TO Q28 OVERLEAF)

Q26 **Thinking of the occasions when you had sexual intercourse in the last 12 months, how often did you use condoms?**
TICK ONE BOX

Always	☐ 1
Most times	☐ 2
About half the time	☐ 3
Occasionally	☐ 4
Never	☐ 5

(14)

Q27 **Now thinking just of the occasions when you have had sexual intercourse with any new partners within the last 12 months, how often did you use a condom?**
TICK ONE BOX

Not had any new partners in last 12 months	☐ 1
Always	☐ 2
Most times	☐ 3
About half the time	☐ 4
Occasionally	☐ 5
Never	☐ 6

(15)

Q28 **Do you intend to use condoms in the next 12 months?**
TICK ONE BOX

Definitely	☐ 1
Probably	☐ 2
Probably not	☐ 3
Definitely not	☐ 4

(16)

Q29 **Have you ever gone on your own initiative to have a blood test for the AIDS virus (HIV test)?**
TICK ONE BOX

No	☐ 1	NOW GO TO Q35
Yes	☐ 2	ANSWER Q30-34

(17)

Q30 **If yes, when was that test? (The last HIV test you have had if more than one.)**
TICK ONE BOX

In the last 12 months	☐ 1
Between 1 and 2 years ago	☐ 2
More than 2 years ago	☐ 3
Can't remember	☐ 4

(18)

Q31 **Why did you go for this HIV test?**
TICK ALL THE BOXES THAT APPLY

Have been at risk of infection through
sexual contact abroad □ 1
Have been at risk of infection through
sexual contact in this country □ 2
Have been at risk of infection through
injecting drug use □ 3

Other reason (PLEASE TICK BOX AND WRITE IN)

. . . . □ 4   (19)

Q32 **And where did you have that test?**
TICK ONE BOX

Blood donor centre □ 1
Ante-natal clinic □ 2
Other hospital department/clinic □ 3
Private doctor or private clinic □ 4
GP or family doctor's surgery/health centre □ 5
STD or VD clinic □ 6
Somewhere else (PLEASE TICK BOX AND WRITE IN WHERE)

. . . . □ 7   (20)

Q33 **Did you receive the results of this test?**
TICK ONE BOX

No □ 1 NOW GO TO Q35
Yes □ 2 ANSWER Q34   (21)

Q34 **How helpful was any counselling you received concerning the HIV test?**
TICK ONE BOX

Did not get any
counselling □ 1
Not at all helpful □ 2
Not very helpful □ 3
Fairly helpful □ 4
Very helpful □ 5   (22)

Q35 **Which of the following applies to you?**
TICK ONE BOX

I have had sexual experience only with males
(or a male), never with a female ☐ 1

I have had sexual experience more often with males,
and at least once with a female ☐ 2

I have had sexual experience about equally often with
males and with females ☐ 3

I have had sexual experience more often with females,
and at least once with a male ☐ 4

I have had sexual experience only with females
(or a female), never with a male ☐ 5

I have never had any sexual experience with anyone ☐ 6 (23)

IF YOU HAVE NEVER HAD ANY SEXUAL EXPERIENCE WITH ANYONE, PLEASE DO
NOT ANSWER ANY FURTHER QUESTIONS (THANKS FOR YOUR HELP). EVERYONE
ELSE PLEASE CONTINUE WITH THE QUESTIONNAIRE.

Q36 **Have you ever had sex with a female involving genital area/vaginal contact?**
TICK ONE BOX

No ☐ 1 GO TO Q38
Yes ☐ 2 ANSWER Q37 (24)

Q37 **If yes, when was the last occasion?**
TICK ONE BOX

Within the last 4 weeks ☐ 1
Between 4 weeks and 3 months ago ☐ 2
Between 3 months and 6 months ago ☐ 3
Between 6 months and 1 year ago ☐ 4
Between 1 year and 5 years ago ☐ 5
More than 5 years ago ☐ 6 (25)

We would now like to ask some questions about your attitudes to condoms. Please remember that **we do need your responses** to these questions, to ensure that we get a representative picture for the whole range of people in this country.

Q38 Listed below are some advantages and disadvantages which people have mentioned about using condoms. Thinking of your own sexual lifestyle and sexual partner(s), please tick **one** box next to each statement to show how likely or unlikely you think it would be in your case.

TICK ONE BOX FOR EACH STATEMENT

	Very unlikely	Fairly unlikely	Fairly likely	Very likely	
Using condoms would...					
...make sex less enjoyable for me	□ 1	□ 2	□ 3	□ 4	(26)
...protect against unwanted pregnancy	□ 1	□ 2	□ 3	□ 4	(27)
...make sex less romantic	□ 1	□ 2	□ 3	□ 4	(28)
...protect against being infected with HIV (the AIDS virus)	□ 1	□ 2	□ 3	□ 4	(29)
...protect against being infected with other sexually transmitted diseases (STDs)	□ 1	□ 2	□ 3	□ 4	(30)
...show that I was a caring person	□ 1	□ 2	□ 3	□ 4	(31)
...make sex less spontaneous	□ 1	□ 2	□ 3	□ 4	(32)
...cause offence to my partner	□ 1	□ 2	□ 3	□ 4	(33)
...make my partner think that I might be infected with HIV	□ 1	□ 2	□ 3	□ 4	(34)
...make me feel less of a woman	□ 1	□ 2	□ 3	□ 4	(35)
...give my partner the impression that I sleep around	□ 1	□ 2	□ 3	□ 4	(36)
...make sex messy	□ 1	□ 2	□ 3	□ 4	(37)
...reduce my sexual pleasure	□ 1	□ 2	□ 3	□ 4	(38)
...reduce my partner's sexual pleasure	□ 1	□ 2	□ 3	□ 4	(39)
...be an annoying interruption to sex	□ 1	□ 2	□ 3	□ 4	(40)
...make sex embarrassing	□ 1	□ 2	□ 3	□ 4	(41)
...be difficult to plan ahead for	□ 1	□ 2	□ 3	□ 4	(42)

Q39 And how much do you care about...
TICK ONE BOX FOR EACH STATEMENT

	Not at all	A little	A lot	
...sex being less enjoyable for you	☐ 1	☐ 2	☐ 3	(43)
...protecting against unwanted pregnancy	☐ 1	☐ 2	☐ 3	(44)
...sex being less romantic	☐ 1	☐ 2	☐ 3	(45)
...protecting against being infected with HIV	☐ 1	☐ 2	☐ 3	(46)
...protecting against being infected with other sexually transmitted diseases	☐ 1	☐ 2	☐ 3	(47)
...showing that you are a caring person	☐ 1	☐ 2	☐ 3	(48)
...sex being less spontaneous	☐ 1	☐ 2	☐ 3	(49)
...causing offence to your partner	☐ 1	☐ 2	☐ 3	(50)
...your partner thinking that you might be infected with HIV	☐ 1	☐ 2	☐ 3	(51)
...feeling less of a woman	☐ 1	☐ 2	☐ 3	(52)
...giving your partner the impression that you sleep around	☐ 1	☐ 2	☐ 3	(53)
...sex being messy	☐ 1	☐ 2	☐ 3	(54)
...your sexual pleasure being reduced	☐ 1	☐ 2	☐ 3	(55)
...your partner's sexual pleasure being reduced	☐ 1	☐ 2	☐ 3	(56)
...having an annoying interruption to sex	☐ 1	☐ 2	☐ 3	(57)
...sex being embarrassing	☐ 1	☐ 2	☐ 3	(58)
...having to plan ahead for sex	☐ 1	☐ 2	☐ 3	(59)

Q40 Listed below are some statements about the views and behaviour of other people. Again, thinking of your sexual lifestyle and sexual partner(s), please tick a box to indicate how much you agree or disagree with each statement.

TICK ONE BOX FOR EACH STATEMENT

	Strongly agree	Tend to agree	Tend to disagree	Strongly disagree	
My current sexual partner thinks we should use condoms	□ 1	□ 2	□ 3	□ 4	(60)
A new sexual partner would want me to use condoms	□ 1	□ 2	□ 3	□ 4	(61)
My friends would approve if I used condoms	□ 1	□ 2	□ 3	□ 4	(62)
My doctor would approve if I used condoms	□ 1	□ 2	□ 3	□ 4	(63)
Government health campaigns recommend that I use condoms	□ 1	□ 2	□ 3	□ 4	(64)
Most people who are important to me would approve if I used condoms	□ 1	□ 2	□ 3	□ 4	(65)

Q41 In general ...

TICK ONE BOX FOR EACH STATEMENT

	Strongly agree	Tend to agree	Tend to disagree	Strongly disagree	
I would want to do what my current sexual partner thinks I should do	□ 1	□ 2	□ 3	□ 4	(66)
I would want to do what a new sexual partner wanted me to do	□ 1	□ 2	□ 3	□ 4	(67)
I would want to do what my friends wanted me to do	□ 1	□ 2	□ 3	□ 4	(68)
I would want to do what my doctor wanted me to do	□ 1	□ 2	□ 3	□ 4	(69)
I would want to do what Government health campaigns recommended me to do	□ 1	□ 2	□ 3	□ 4	(70)

Q42 **How likely is it that each of the following would stop you using condoms, even if you wished to use them?**
TICK ONE BOX FOR EACH STATEMENT

	Very unlikely	Fairly unlikely	Fairly likely	Very likely	
Feeling embarrassed to buy condoms	☐ 1	☐ 2	☐ 3	☐ 4	(71)
Forgetting to carry them with you	☐ 1	☐ 2	☐ 3	☐ 4	(72)
Difficulty in using a condom	☐ 1	☐ 2	☐ 3	☐ 4	(73)
The cost of condoms	☐ 1	☐ 2	☐ 3	☐ 4	(74)
Difficulty in obtaining condoms	☐ 1	☐ 2	☐ 3	☐ 4	(75)
Getting carried away in the heat of the moment	☐ 1	☐ 2	☐ 3	☐ 4	(76)
Difficulty in talking about using condoms	☐ 1	☐ 2	☐ 3	☐ 4	(77)
Your partner getting angry if you suggested using condoms	☐ 1	☐ 2	☐ 3	☐ 4	(78)
Fear of giving a bad impression about your own sexual behaviour if you suggested using condoms	☐ 1	☐ 2	☐ 3	☐ 4	(79)
Difficulty in planning ahead for sex	☐ 1	☐ 2	☐ 3	☐ 4	(80)

CARD ⑪ :0

Q43 **How strongly do you agree or disagree with each of these statements?**
TICK ONE BOX FOR EACH STATEMENT

	Strongly agree	Tend to agree	Tend to disagree	Strongly disagree	
For me, the disadvantages of using condoms would outweigh the advantages	☐ 1	☐ 2	☐ 3	☐ 4	(11)
For me, using condoms would be a good idea	☐ 1	☐ 2	☐ 3	☐ 4	(12)
Most people whose opinions I value think I should use condoms	☐ 1	☐ 2	☐ 3	☐ 4	(13)
I intend to use condoms in the future	☐ 1	☐ 2	☐ 3	☐ 4	(14)
More and more people are using condoms these days	☐ 1	☐ 2	☐ 3	☐ 4	(15)
More and more of my friends are using condoms these days	☐ 1	☐ 2	☐ 3	☐ 4	(16)

Q44 How much control do you have over whether or not you use condoms?
TICK ONE BOX

Complete control	A lot of control	Some control	Very little control
☐ 1	☐ 2	☐ 3	☐ 4 (17)

Q45 How easy or difficult would it be for you to do each of the following, if you wanted to?
TICK ONE BOX FOR EACH ITEM

	Very easy	Fairly easy	Fairly difficult	Very difficult
Choose sexual partners that were not at risk of infection	☐ 1	☐ 2	☐ 3	☐ 4 (18)
Use condoms with a sexual partner	☐ 1	☐ 2	☐ 3	☐ 4 (19)
Persuade a sexual partner to have sex with a condom if they didn't want to	☐ 1	☐ 2	☐ 3	☐ 4 (20)

Thinking of the next 12 months . . . .

Q46 **How likely is it that you will use condoms in the next 12 months?**
TICK ONE BOX

Very unlikely	Fairly unlikely	Fairly likely	Very likely	
☐ 1	☐ 2	☐ 3	☐ 4	(21)

Q47 **Thinking of the occasions when you may have sexual intercourse in the next 12 months, how often do you think you will use condoms?**
TICK ONE BOX

Always	Most times	About half the time	Occasionally	Never	
☐ 1	☐ 2	☐ 3	☐ 4	☐ 5	(22)

Q48 **How likely is it that you would use condoms if you had sex with a new partner?**
TICK ONE BOX

Very unlikely	Fairly unlikely	Fairly likely	Very likely	
☐ 1	☐ 2	☐ 3	☐ 4	(23)

Q49 **Thinking just of the occasions when you may have sexual intercourse with any new partners in the next 12 months, how often do you think you will use condoms?**
TICK ONE BOX

Always	Most times	About half the time	Occasionally	Never	
☐ 1	☐ 2	☐ 3	☐ 4	☐ 5	(24)

THANK YOU VERY MUCH FOR COMPLETING THIS QUESTIONNAIRE

YOUR ANSWERS WILL BE KEPT IN COMPLETE CONFIDENCE

Appendix B. Weighting matrix

Region	Men 16–19	20–24	25–34	35–44	45–54	55–74	Women 16–19	20–24	25–34	35–44	45–54	55–74
01	0.202	0.306	0.696	0.592	0.552	0.817	0.193	0.305	0.688	0.577	0.548	0.922
02	0.256	0.385	0.823	0.712	0.656	0.939	0.241	0.374	0.825	0.700	0.645	1.048
03	0.317	0.494	1.117	0.927	0.860	1.245	0.297	0.480	1.086	0.903	0.846	1.355
04	0.163	0.245	0.533	0.457	0.428	0.615	0.157	0.241	0.533	0.456	0.429	0.696
05	0.274	0.423	0.916	0.783	0.721	1.003	0.266	0.410	0.900	0.753	0.701	1.132
06	0.366	0.552	1.196	1.015	0.961	1.376	0.340	0.529	1.158	0.982	0.936	1.487
07	0.196	0.305	0.659	0.519	0.462	0.614	0.178	0.278	0.628	0.530	0.465	0.659
08	0.219	0.338	0.686	0.549	0.504	0.792	0.199	0.300	0.643	0.568	0.529	0.903
09	0.228	0.340	0.712	0.657	0.636	0.909	0.212	0.330	0.711	0.627	0.591	1.030
10	0.148	0.232	0.473	0.387	0.365	0.564	0.138	0.213	0.465	0.399	0.364	0.613
11	0.135	0.229	0.471	0.380	0.351	0.473	0.131	0.221	0.466	0.392	0.352	0.505
12	0.106	0.180	0.370	0.298	0.276	0.372	0.103	0.173	0.366	0.308	0.277	0.397
13	0.155	0.267	0.551	0.443	0.405	0.568	0.151	0.266	0.549	0.450	0.408	0.620
14	0.099	0.170	0.352	0.283	0.259	0.363	0.097	0.170	0.351	0.288	0.261	0.396
15	0.085	0.132	0.282	0.242	0.226	0.321	0.080	0.128	0.279	0.243	0.229	0.362
16	0.118	0.182	0.163	0.335	0.312	0.443	0.110	0.176	0.385	0.336	0.316	0.500
17	0.092	0.151	0.309	0.259	0.237	0.349	0.088	0.147	0.301	0.256	0.238	0.396
18	0.157	0.257	0.526	0.441	0.403	0.594	0.151	0.250	0.513	0.437	0.404	0.675
Total	3.32	5.188	10.835	9.279	8.610	12.358	3.130	4.993	10.848	9.205	8.539	13.696
												100.00

(Base: All)

Those completing the sexual behaviour booklet

Region	Men					Women				
	16–19	20–24	25–34	35–44	45–54	16–19	20–24	25–34	35–44	45–54
01	0.274	0.414	0.941	0.801	0.746	0.261	0.413	0.931	0.780	0.741
02	0.346	0.520	1.112	0.963	0.887	0.327	0.505	1.116	0.946	0.872
03	0.428	0.668	1.510	1.253	1.163	0.401	0.649	1.469	1.221	1.144
04	0221	0.331	0.721	0.617	0.578	0.212	0.326	0.721	0.616	0.580
05	0.371	0.572	1.239	1.059	0.975	0.360	0.555	1.216	1.018	0.948
06	0.495	0.747	1.618	1.373	1.299	0.460	0.716	1.566	1.328	1.266
07	0.264	0.413	0.892	0.702	0.625	0.241	0.376	0.849	0.717	0.629
08	0.297	0.457	0.927	0.742	0.681	0.269	0.406	0.870	0.768	0.716
09	0.309	0.460	0.963	0.888	0.860	0.286	0.447	0.962	0.847	0.799
10	0.200	0.314	0.639	0.524	0.493	0.186	0.288	0.629	0.540	0.492
11	0.182	0.310	0.637	0.514	0.474	0.177	0.298	0.630	0.530	0.477
12	0.143	0.243	0.500	0.404	0.373	0.139	0.235	0.495	0.416	0.374
13	0.210	0.361	0.745	0.599	0.547	0.204	0.360	0.743	0.609	0.551
14	0.134	0.230	0.476	0.383	0.350	0.131	0.230	0.475	0.389	0.352
15	0.116	0.178	0.381	0.328	0.306	0.108	0.173	0.377	0.329	0.310
16	0.160	0.246	0.221	0.453	0.422	0.149	0.238	0.521	0.455	0.428
17	0.125	0.204	0.418	0.350	0.320	0.120	0.199	0.407	0.347	0.321
18	0.213	0.348	0.712	0.596	0.545	0.204	0.338	0.694	0.590	0.547
Total	4.488	7.016	14.653	12.549	11.644	4.233	6.753	14.670	12.448	11.548
100.000	0.000	0.000	0.000	0.000	0.000	0.000	0.000	0.000	0.000	0.000

(Excludes 55–74)